ncw
10/4/13.
616.
075
JOH

The Minor Illness Manual

FOURTH EDITION

Minor Illness Specialist Nurse; Emergency Nurse Practitioner;
Nurse Independent Prescriber

Foreword by

PROFESSOR SUE CROSS

Primary Care Nursing, London South Bank University
Advisor to HMP Bedford and London-wide Local Medical Committees

Radcliffe Publishing
London • New York

Radcliffe Publishing Ltd
33–41 Dallington Street
London
EC1V 0BB
United Kingdom

www.radcliffepublishing.com

© 2012 Gina Johnson and Ian Hill-Smith

First Edition 1997
Second Edition 2000
Third Edition 2006

Gina Johnson and Ian Hill-Smith have asserted their right under the Copyright, Designs and Patents Act 1988 to be identified as the authors of this work.

British Library Cataloguing in Publication Data

A catalogue record for this book is available from the British Library.

ISBN-13: 978 184619 564 8

The paper used for the text pages of this book is FSC® certified. FSC (The Forest Stewardship Council®) is an international network to promote responsible management of the world's forests.

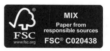

Typeset by Darkriver Design, Auckland, New Zealand
Printed and bound by Hobbs the Printers, Totton, Hants, UK

Contents

Foreword to the fourth edition

It is good to see the next edition of *The Minor Illness Manual* on the shelves, although I am sure that most of the patients with the conditions covered in this book don't consider them as minor! When I started in practice nursing over 20 years ago, the minor illnesses that were the responsibility of the nurse were restricted to coughs, colds and the occasional sore throat. Now the role of the nurse in all areas of primary care has grown dramatically, and the level of knowledge and skills required are far greater than mine in those early days; therefore, it is paramount that we have excellent resources to enable us to keep up to date.

To support the advanced education that nurses need, we require equally advanced sources of reliable information on current practice. This enables us to maintain the high quality of care which we strive to give our patients. Therefore, the present edition of this book comes at exactly the right time.

There are enormous political changes afoot, as we are all aware, but these can lead to exciting opportunities for all health professionals in primary care to extend and develop their roles in ways that were unheard of a few years ago.

I congratulate the authors on their excellent work, which ensures that all clinicians who manage the conditions covered in this book can have accessible, up-to-date and evidence-based guidelines to support their work in primary care.

Professor Sue Cross
Primary Care Nursing, London South Bank University
Advisor to HMP Bedford and London-wide Local Medical Committees
October 2011

Preface to the fourth edition

The National Health Service (NHS) is again in a state of turbulent change, with clinical commissioning groups gearing up to take over the roles of primary care trusts and strategic health authorities. Instability, which is becoming a rare constant within the NHS, together with uncertainty about the role of private companies in providing healthcare, undermines confidence in future employment for a wide range of healthcare professionals. Traditional boundaries between professions are being swept away, as nurses take on more diagnosis and treatment, pharmacists advise on an expanding range of medication available on or off prescription, and doctors are finding challenges from their new commissioning responsibilities. Labels are of little help. Job descriptions such as 'emergency care practitioner' or 'nurse practitioner' are open to interpretation; such posts may be filled by colleagues with widely varying backgrounds. It has never been more important to focus on your area of expertise and to develop it in a way that will be both rewarding for you and useful to future patients.

Nurses are now taking responsibility for managing more serious acute infections; for example, community matrons are treating pyelonephritis, Urgent Care Centre nurses are prescribing oral steroids for croup, and minor illness specialists in general practice are managing acute exacerbations of asthma and chronic obstructive pulmonary disease. We have therefore extended the scope of this manual to cover these conditions, with the caveat that they should only be managed by nurses with appropriate experience.

The Department of Health is keen to encourage 'self-care', which is considered one of the key components of a patient-centred health service. We have responded by identifying and expanding the advice on self-care in each section of the book, and by extending the range of topics to include recommendations on ailments where the evidence on appropriate management is hard to find. Medications available without a prescription are clearly identified in the formulary section.

The key skills needed to manage minor illness have not changed: the ability to uncover and address the patient's agenda, to relieve distressing symptoms and to identify the small proportion of people who have serious disease as promptly as possible.

Gina Johnson
Ian Hill-Smith
October 2011

v

About the editors and contributors

National Minor Illness Centre (NMIC)
All of the authors work together in Kingfisher Practice, an NHS general practice near Luton Airport. Previously known as Stopsley Group Practice, it is a research and training practice which cares for nearly 8000 patients. In 1996, the practice designed an innovative educational programme for nurses on the management of minor illness, and in 2007 the National Minor Illness Centre was developed as an educational component to the practice. By September 2011, over 1000 nurses had attended NMIC seminar weeks, the majority of whom achieved university accreditation.

Dr Gina Johnson graduated from Guy's Hospital in London in 1979 and has worked as a general practitioner in Luton since 1983. She has always been actively involved in primary care audit and research, and has published articles on a wide range of topics. She is very aware of the limitations of Western medicine, which led her to study for an MSc in medical anthropology in 2002. She is a medical acupuncturist, and has an interest in holistic care.

Ian Hill-Smith started publishing research papers while studying for his first degree in anatomy, before graduating in medicine from University College, London, in 1980. He is both a member of the Royal College of Physicians and a fellow of the Royal College of General Practitioners. He is fascinated by fundamental science and how it can be applied to medical practice, particularly how medicines can be prescribed to best effect (which was the subject of his research MD). He chairs the Luton Primary Care Prescribing Committee, and has developed a successful training course on medicines management.

Amber Kelly moved from health visiting to practice nursing and then gained qualifications in family planning, diabetes nursing and teaching, and a degree in community nursing. She trained as a nurse independent prescriber while completing minor illness training, and has designed and published nursing research. Her greatest personal growth came from attaining a degree in literature and historical studies and on achieving a master's degree in literature.

Rosemary Brand trained at Barts, qualifying in 1975. She worked in South Africa, qualified as a midwife, and then spent 25 years in accident and emergency departments in Jersey, York, Newport and Watford. She worked at Luton Walk-in Centre for 4 years before joining Kingfisher Practice in 2007, bringing a new dimension to the team.

Acknowledgements

We would like to thank our staff at the Kingfisher Practice for their ongoing support. The practice has recently been through a period of transition, and without the exceptional skills and dedication of our practice manager, Lindsay Reyner, this edition would never have been written. We would also like to thank our own highly skilled minor illness nurses, both past and present (especially Rhona Rollings), our stalwart partner Sarah Burcombe, and our previous partner Chris Ellis.

We are grateful to the many nurses and paramedics who have attended our courses and seminars, who have taught us so much. Thanks are also due to Luton community pharmacist Farwaj Chaudhuri for his invaluable input.

We acknowledge the excellent work of the Prodigy team (previously Clinical Knowledge Summaries) in gathering together the evidence for the management of a wide range of conditions, and would like to thank them for their patience in responding to our queries and comments.

We also thank our patients, for allowing us to learn from their experiences of minor illness.

The nurses' perspective on changes and safe practice in primary care

AMBER KELLY, ROSEMARY BRAND

Nurse practitioners, advanced nurse practitioners, community matrons, rapid response teams, nurse independent prescribers, minor illness and other specialist nurses have all had a positive impact on the public's perception of nurses working at higher levels of practice in primary care. Working in walk-in centres, urgent care centres, general practices, out-of-hours services, NHS Direct and across the community setting, nurse-led care is evident and thriving. Many practice nurses are also working as minor illness specialist nurses, as the first point of contact for patients presenting in general practice who request same-day appointments. In 2009, 56% of GP practices had minor illness nurses.[1] Some patients are unable to name their GPs, as their only contact with health professionals in general practice are the nurses who assess, diagnose and recommend or prescribe treatment for their presenting ailments. In terms of cost-effectiveness, nurses represent exceptional value for money, undertaking roles that were traditionally those of doctors at a fraction of the cost. With 57 million GP consultations every year involving a minor ailment, and 91% of them ending in a prescription, the cost to the NHS is £2 billion. This cost is mainly for GPs' time.[2]

The greatest facilitator to higher levels of practice and nurse autonomy has been the move into non-medical prescribing. It is one of the biggest changes to happen to the profession of nursing, and has benefited patients through quicker access to treatment and in continuity of care. Nurse independent prescribers (NIPs) are able to prescribe from the entire *British National Formulary*, including unlicensed medicines, as can supplementary prescribers (providing clinical management plans are in place). Training for NIP (V200 and V300) in England is delivered over 6 months, to degree level, at institutes of higher education. A limited nurse prescribers' formulary for community practitioners is available to health visitors and district nurses as part of their training (V100) and it is also offered as a stand-alone prescribing course (V150). In May 2011, the number of nurse prescribers with effective registration were:

- Community Practitioner Nurse Prescriber (V100) – 33 033
- Community Practitioner Nurse Prescriber (V150) – 728

- Nurse Independent Prescriber (V200) – 1526
- Nurse Independent/Supplementary Prescriber (V300) – 21 976[3]

Nurse prescribers have proved to be safe, prescribing only within their own competencies. Minor illness nurses who prescribe frequently and with the aid of a computer often become more confident than nurses who have to hand-write occasional prescriptions. Computer software is used in general practice to facilitate prescribing in consultations, linking patients' records to drug interactions and contraindications. In circumstances where a minor illness nurse does not hold a registered prescribing qualification, and is assessing patients and recommending necessary treatments by generating a prescription, a GP must sign the prescription and take responsibility for it. Appropriate professional indemnity is essential, especially for prescribers. For nurses working in general practice and for private employers, the Medical Defence Union and the Medical Protection Society (or similar organisations) have group schemes to cover both the general practitioners and the nurses employed by them.

The minor illness specialist course that accompanies this manual has been running since 1996. To date, over 1000 nurses have attended the course, which runs over 6 months, starting with 5 days of seminars followed by 6 months of clinical sessions at the student's workplace, and successful completion of assignments. It is accredited by the University of Bedfordshire for 45 credits at Level 3. The course can be attended without accreditation, but it is education and training that ultimately define fitness for practice. A certificate of attendance is given to those nurses attending the seminars and not undertaking accreditation, but is not proof of competence in the management of minor illness. A formal assessment, incorporated into a period of practice with a designated medical supervisor, is essential to demonstrate the ability to apply theory to practice. This should be followed by a signed certificate stating the nurse's competence to manage minor illness that should be retained as evidence of competence. As the Nursing and Midwifery Council (NMC) code (2008) states:

- You must have the knowledge and skills for safe and effective practice when working without direct supervision.
- You must recognise and work within the limits of your competence.[4]

All nurses are familiar with the concept of legal and professional accountability. Accountability for practice, knowledge and competence lies ultimately with the registered nurse as embedded in the NMC code.

Once underpinned by education and training, *The Minor Illness Manual* offers guidelines to support decision making in the management of conditions commonly presenting in primary care. These guidelines can be used to enable safe and effective practice. In individual GP practices, any guidelines should be mutually agreed upon by the GPs and the minor illness nurses. Where there are discrepancies, perhaps regarding local variations in antimicrobial treatment or disagreement regarding treatment, revised guidelines should be written and documented. If a nurse, for whatever reason, then works outside the agreed remit, she needs to document on whose authority this was done. Elsewhere in primary care (and especially in nurse-led services), nurses will often be required to adhere to more rigid protocols and more extensive documentation. This 'defensive' stance of nurses often mystifies and frustrates medical practitioners, who feel secure in their positions, while nurses may feel vulnerable in theirs.

Increased responsibility brings increased stress, inherent with extended nursing roles and higher levels of practice. Any move into higher levels of practice should be accompanied by increased remuneration. GPs are independent employers, and practice nurses, as GP employees, do not have equitable pay and conditions. They also experience disparity with other NHS colleagues. Research undertaken into prescribing among practice nurses in Bedfordshire[5] showed few GP practices had adopted *Agenda for Change*, and it identified lack of wages as a barrier to the intention to train in prescribing. It also recommended realistic financial incentives for professional development, and that GPs consult their nurse employees over the adoption of *Agenda for Change* to ensure parity of pay and conditions with other NHS colleagues. It is widely recognised among nurses that non-medical prescribing carries a potential risk to their registration, despite awareness of accountability and the code of conduct which defines nursing practice. Nurses will always be more conscious of this risk than their employers.[6] It is essential for employers to provide time to access clinical supervision, either formally or informally, in order to combat any stress, and it should be timetabled into the working week.

Continuing professional development is integral to safe and effective practice and as evidence of competence. It does not always have to be accessed through formal courses, workshops or study days. In order to keep updated in minor illness management, the National Minor Illness Centre (NMIC) website at www.minorillness.co.uk has a members' section which is open to all health professionals for an annual fee. This section, amongst other benefits, provides access to e-learning resources. Crucially, it sends e-mail alerts when there is an important change in prescribing and management of any minor illness. All alerts are the latest evidence-based information and are sent in order to promote and improve standards in the delivery of patient care.

On its troubled passage to legislation, the Health and Social Care Bill (2011)[7] has already been hailed as the biggest restructure of the NHS since its inception. When it becomes law, primary care trusts (PCTs) and strategic health authorities (SHAs) will be abolished. The bill proposed a GP-managed NHS with GP commissioning consortia holding up to 80% of the NHS budget. Professional and political outcry led to establishment of the NHS Future Forum,[8] the government's 'listening exercise' committee reviewing the Health and Social Care Bill. An amendment to the bill has been passed, with the majority of the NHS budget and the commissioning of services to be placed with multidisciplinary clinical commissioning groups (CCGs) from both the primary and secondary sectors. Nurses will have places on commissioning boards, which should influence the provision of future funding for the continuing increase in nurse-led services. At the time of this edition of *The Minor Illness Manual*, the Health and Social Care Bill has still some distance to go before becoming law. Some nurses are already involved as members of local commissioning boards, and many hold the necessary leadership skills to become involved in commissioning healthcare and contribute to the future funding and delivery of nurse-led services. Skill mix is essential on local boards for informed decision making in service development. Decommissioning will also be on the agenda, with the NHS expected to save some £20 billion over the next 4 years. Nurses represent excellent value for money as they move further into roles that were the traditional domain of doctors.

The first *Minor Illness Manual* appeared in 1997, when the notion of a nurse-led service in general practice appeared radical. Now in its fourth edition, it has sold more than 20 000 copies, testimony to the growth, acceptance (by patients and medical staff) and success of higher-level nursing in the delivery of healthcare in a rapidly changing NHS.

References

1   TNS Healthcare. *Making the Case for the Self-Care of Minor Ailments*. Commissioned by the Proprietary Association of Great Britain. 2009. Available at: www.pagb.co.uk/information/PDFs/Minorailmentsresearch09.pdf (accessed 6 April 2011).

2   Ibid.

3   Personal communication from Records and Archives Department, Nursing and Midwifery Council, 2 May 2011.

4   Nursing and Midwifery Council. *The Code: standards of conduct, performance and ethics for nurses and midwives*. London: Nursing and Midwifery Council; 2008.

5   Kelly A, Neale J, Rollings R. Barriers to extended nurse prescribing among practice nurses. *Community Pract*. 2010; **83**(1): 21–4.

6   [No author listed]. Letter to the editor. *Nurse Prescribing*. 2011; **9**: 5.

7   Department of Health. *The Health and Social Care Bill*. 2011. Available at: www.publications.parliament.uk/pa/cmbills/132/en/1132en.htm (accessed 27 March 2011).

8   Department of Health. *NHS Future Forum Publishes Recommendations to Government*. 2011 http://healthandcare.dh.gov.uk/future-forum-report (accessed 14 July 2011).

Introduction

General advice

History
- listening is the greatest skill. What is the patient's agenda?
- open questions may reveal hidden concerns
- most diagnoses are made on the history – 'listen to the patient: he is telling you the diagnosis'

Examination
- this may reveal important signs, but will also serve to reassure the patient

Tests
- only useful if the management depends on the result
- may give false positive results and cause unnecessary concern

Self-care
- discuss the options, and agree the proposed plan of management with the patient
- worsening advice: ask the patient to contact the most appropriate NHS service if the situation worsens or there is no improvement within a specified time

Prescription/antibiotics
- *see* Formulary for prescribing information, page 153

Caution
- although guidelines support clinical judgement, they can never replace experience and intuition

High-risk groups for infections

Immunosuppressed
- due to *medication*: e.g. prednisolone, azathioprine, disease-modifying anti-rheumatic drugs (DMARDs) such as methotrexate, ciclosporin, cyclophosphamide, recent chemotherapy
- due to *medical conditions* which reduce the immune response: e.g. human immunodeficiency virus (HIV), leukaemia, diabetes, splenectomy, malnutrition, pregnancy, prematurity, inherited immunodeficiency

Long-term conditions
- significant heart, lung, kidney, liver or neuromuscular disease

National Institute for Health and Clinical Excellence (NICE), 2008

1

Fever and flu-like illness

Fever

Sometimes fever alone is the presenting problem. A careful history will usually identify the likely source, but sometimes this is not obvious. Be aware that although most patients with a flu-like illness will indeed have a simple viral infection, there are many uncommon diseases which can cause the same initial symptoms. Ask open questions to see if there could be an alternative source of infection (such as the urinary tract). This is particularly important if the history has some odd features, or if the symptoms have been present for more than 5 days. For more information on fever in children, *see* page 10.

History
- duration
- rigors (suggest bacterial infection)
- joint and muscle pains
- sore throat
- headache
- vomiting/diarrhoea
- cough
- rash (other viral infections, toxic shock, septicaemia?)
- urinary symptoms (pyelonephritis?)
- possibility of pregnancy
- lactating (mastitis?)
- travel to tropical region in last 12 months (malaria, or other tropical disease?)
- exposure to rats' urine (e.g. in sewers or rivers – risk of leptospirosis)
- high-risk group (*see* page 6)

Examination (modified as suggested by symptoms)
- temperature (taking into account any recent antipyretic)
- pulse rate
- respiratory rate
- blood pressure in adults

- capillary refill time (CRT) in children
- oxygen saturation, if serious illness suspected
- ears
- throat
- cervical lymph nodes
- chest
- rash (beware the petechial rash of meningitis)
- neck or back stiffness (e.g. can a child kiss his knees?)
- breasts, in lactating women
- any painful area (e.g. abdomen)

Tests

- test urine for nitrites, leucocytes and blood if cause of fever not obvious (to avoid contaminating the whole sample, pour a little urine on the test strip)
- send mid-stream urine (MSU) for culture if test positive, or any urinary symptoms
- if travel to tropical area in last 12 months, thick and thin blood film and full blood count (FBC). If the first test is negative, repeat the blood film after 12–24 h. If the second test is negative, repeat the blood film again after a further 24 h

Self-care

- adequate fluid intake
- avoid over-strenuous activity
- paracetamol or ibuprofen, only if needed to relieve discomfort
- assume a viral cause if no other clues, fever less than 5 days' duration and generally well
- otherwise give treatment appropriate to cause
- reduce anxiety about fever by explaining that it is produced by the body's immune system in response to an infection, is unlikely to cause any harm and may aid recovery
- advice on what to do if symptoms worsen: 'worsening advice'

Refer to doctor

- immediately if:
  - temperature of ≥ 38°C in a baby under 3 months or a temperature of ≥ 39°C in a baby under 6 months
  - photophobia, neck stiffness, drowsiness or petechial rash
  - severe illness
  - prostration (unable to stand up)
  - unexplained fever lasting more than 5 days
  - risk of leptospirosis
  - immunosuppressed

Cautions

- mastitis may cause flu-like symptoms in a breastfeeding woman with only minimal signs in the breast
- malaria may cause an illness indistinguishable from flu, and taking malaria prophylaxis may not prevent malaria. If patient has visited an area where falciparum malaria occurs,

a 'test and treat' strategy is recommended where empirical treatment is given without waiting for the test result

- meningitis in its early stages is impossible to distinguish from a simple viral infection. Diarrhoea and vomiting may cause confusion with gastro-enteritis, and the rash of meningococcal septicaemia may initially appear macular and blanch on pressure
- persistent fever with no associated other symptoms or signs of a focus of infection may require thorough investigation in hospital to discover the hidden cause

References

National Institute for Health and Clinical Excellence. *Feverish Illness in Children: assessment and initial management in children younger than 5 years*. NICE guideline 47. London: NIHCE; 2007. www.nice.org.uk/guidance/CG47

Thompson MJ, Ninis N, Perera R, *et al*. Clinical recognition of meningococcal disease in children and adolescents. *Lancet*. 2006; **367**(9508): 397–493. doi: 10.1016/S0140-6736(06)67932–4.

Flu-like illness

History

- onset – sudden or gradual?
- duration
- fever
- joint and muscle pains
- sore throat
- headache
- vomiting/diarrhoea
- productive cough
- rash (other viral infections, septicaemia?)
- possibility of pregnancy
- high-risk group (*see* page 6)

Examination

- temperature (taking into account any recent antipyretic)
- pulse
- respiratory rate
- throat
- chest
- in seriously ill adults, blood pressure (BP) and oxygen saturation
- in seriously ill children, capillary refill time (CRT) and oxygen saturation

Tests

- urinalysis (if rigors or urinary symptoms)

Self-care

- paracetamol or ibuprofen as required for sore throat and headache

- ensure adequate fluid intake
- 'worsening advice'

Prescription
- antiviral medicines (oseltamivir, zanamavir) may be indicated if there is a recognized flu epidemic. They shorten the duration of the illness by less than 1 day, but reduce the risk of complications (to what extent is contentious). See www.hpa.org.uk for current advice

Refer to doctor
- urgently for possible hospital admission if:
  — temperature of ≥ 38°C in a baby under 3 months or a temperature of ≥ 39°C in a baby under 6 months
  — severe illness – the patient seems more ill than you would expect
  — prostration (unable to stand up)
  — dehydrated
  — respiratory rate above 50/min under 1 year, 40/min under 6, 30/min or more age 6–adult
  — systolic BP of 90 mmHg or less, or diastolic BP of 60 mmHg or less in adults
  — CRT ≥ 3 s in children
  — oxygen saturation below 95%
  — fever lasting more than 5 days

Reference
Prodigy. *Clinical topic: Influenza – seasonal.* 2011. Available at: http://prodigy.clarity.co.uk/ influenza_seasonal (accessed 29 August 2011).

Feverish illness in children under five

We recommend that you carefully study the summary of this NICE (2007) guideline, which provides a framework for the assessment of feverish children. We would like to draw your attention to the following points:

1 The routine assessment of a feverish child should include:
  - temperature (taken with an axillary thermometer in babies under 4 weeks)
  - heart rate
  - respiratory rate
  - capillary refill time

2 A temperature of ≥ 38°C in a baby under 3 months or a temperature of ≥ 39°C in a baby under 6 months is an indication for hospital assessment.

3 The routine use of medicines for the sole purpose of lowering fever is to be discouraged, in particular the use of ibuprofen and paracetamol at the same time. There is no evidence that antipyretic medicines can prevent febrile convulsions, and there is evidence from animal studies that their use may increase mortality in influenza.

References

Eyers S, Weatherall M, Shirtcliffe P, *et al*. The effect on mortality of antipyretics in the treatment of influenza infection: systematic review and meta-analysis. *J Roy Soc Med*. 2010; **103**: 403–11.

National Institute for Health and Clinical Excellence. *Feverish Illness in Children: assessment and initial management in children younger than 5 years. NICE guideline 47*. London: NIHCE; 2007. www.nice.org.uk/guidance/CG47

Prymula R, Siegrist CA, Chlibek R, *et al*. Effect of prophylactic paracetamol administration at time of vaccination on febrile reactions and antibody responses in children: two open-label, randomised controlled trials. *Lancet*. 2009; **374**: 1339–50.

Sullivan JE, Farrar HC, Section on Clinical Pharmacology and Therapeutics, *et al*. Clinical report: fever and antipyretic use in children. *Pediatrics*. 2011; doi: 10.1542/peds.2010–3852.

TABLE 1.1 Assessment of the feverish child under five (NICE, 2007)

	Green – low risk	Amber – intermediate risk	Red – high risk
Colour	• normal colour of skin, lips and tongue	• pallor reported by parent/carer	• pale/mottled/ashen/blue
Activity	• responds normally to social cues • content/smiles • stays awake or awakens quickly • strong normal cry/not crying	• not responding normally to social cues • wakes only with prolonged stimulation • decreased activity • no smile	• no response to social cues • appears ill to a healthcare professional • unable to rouse or if roused does not stay awake • weak, high-pitched or continuous cry

Respiratory	• normal	• nasal flaring
		• tachypnoea:
		  • RR > 50 breaths/minute age 6–12 months
		  • RR > 40 breaths/minute age > 12 months
		• oxygen saturation ≤ 95% in air
		• crackles
			• grunting
			• tachypnoea:
			  • RR > 60 breaths/minute
			• moderate or severe chest indrawing or recession

Hydration	• normal skin and eyes • moist mucous membranes	• dry mucous membrane • poor feeding in infants • CRT ≥ 3 seconds • reduced urine output	• reduced skin turgor
Other	• *none* of the amber or red symptoms or signs	• fever for ≥ 5 days • swelling of a limb or joint • non-weight bearing/not using an extremity • a new lump > 2 cm	• age 0–3 months, temperature ≥ 38°C • age 3–6 months, temperature ≥ 39°C • non-blanching rash • bulging fontanelle • neck stiffness • status epilepticus • focal neurological signs • focal seizures • bile-stained vomiting

CRT, capillary refill time; RR, respiratory rate.

Serious bacterial infection in adults and older children

- these conditions are rare in primary care
- the early stages of meningitis and septicaemia may be indistinguishable from flu
- consider if patient very unwell with fever and drowsiness
- headache, prostration, photophobia
- rigors (suggest urinary cause)
- cold mottled extremities, maybe cyanosis
- severe joint and muscle pain
- abdominal pain, maybe diarrhoea and vomiting
- reduced urine output
- rapid pulse and respiration
- low BP
- check carefully for a rash. In the early stages of meningococcal infection a rash is not always present, and may not be purpuric
- sometimes you will not be able to make the diagnosis
- careful examination, explanation and record-keeping are your best safeguards
- if in any doubt, explain warning signs, advise patient to have someone with them who will check them regularly

2

Respiratory tract infections

Acute cough

History
- duration
- dry/productive/wheezy
- hoarseness
- colour of sputum, if bloodstained
- fever
- chest pain
- breathlessness
- previous similar episodes (how treated and what happened)
- smoking (amount, duration)
- high-risk group

Examination
- temperature
- cyanosis
- respiratory rate
- breathlessness
- subcostal/intercostal recession (especially in babies)
- crackles in chest (and where located)
- quality of breath sounds
- percussion
- wheezing
- in sick adults, BP and pulse
- in sick children, capillary refill time

Tests
- peak flow rate if wheezing heard in adult or child over 7 years (*see* section on acute asthma, page 21)
- oxygen saturation

- sputum culture is unhelpful, except in special cases: cystic fibrosis, bronchiectasis, persistent purulent sputum in chronic obstructive pulmonary disease (COPD), or suspected tuberculosis
- consider chest X-ray in smokers or if sputum bloodstained

Specific types of cough

Cough is a very common problem; other symptoms may accompany it and help to make a diagnosis. The patient may seek help because the cough is persistent or interferes with sleep, or because of anxiety that infection is 'going to the chest'. Quite often a friend or relative has suggested that the patient should seek medical help. Mothers may fear that their children will choke in the night.

Acute cough (less than 3 weeks' duration) may be due to:
- upper respiratory tract infections, e.g. common cold (viral)
- acute bronchitis (usually viral)
- acute laryngitis (viral), associated with hoarseness
- pneumonia (viral or bacterial)
- croup in children (viral)
- bronchiolitis in children (viral)
- exacerbations of asthma (viral)
- exacerbations of COPD or bronchiectasis (bacterial)
- physical and chemical stimuli, e.g. cold air, cigarette smoke
- pulmonary embolism; unilateral pleuritic chest pain, dry cough, dyspnoea and sometimes haemoptysis

A persistent or relapsing cough may occur in:
- post-viral cough, which may last for several weeks. Patients may expect proprietary cough medicines to cure the cough, and come for something stronger because brand X 'hasn't worked'. They need gentle re-education. Cough medicines for 'chesty coughs' (expectorants) exacerbate cough!
- angiotensin-converting enzyme inhibitor (ACEI) therapy (drug names ending in -pril)
- heart failure may cause a persistent cough, with fine crackles at both lung bases
- pertussis (whooping cough)
- *Mycoplasma pneumoniae*, an unusual type of infection which occurs in cycles of 3–5 years. It causes a cough which may last for 3 months. It is sensitive to clarithromycin or doxycycline, but not amoxicillin. A 2-week course is necessary
- tuberculosis
- asthma (young children may present with cough without wheezing)
- heavy smokers (but beware cancer)
- allergic rhinitis
- acid reflux
- lung cancer. A persistent cough in a smoker, associated with chest pain, haemoptysis or weight loss, is suspicious
- habit

Self-care

- most acute coughs due to the common cold or acute bronchitis; although acute bronchitis may sometimes be caused by bacteria, antibiotics provide little benefit in these conditions unless there is co-morbidity
- adequate fluid intake
- stop smoking (includes parents of coughing child)
- soothing drinks, e.g. manuka honey and lemon
- some people find linctuses helpful, e.g. simple linctus
- menthol, either inhaled or in a linctus, has a short-lived cough suppressant effect
- chocolate (contains theobromine) and alcohol may help – maybe liqueur chocolates?
- pelargonium extract (Kaloba) has been shown in two trials to reduce sputum production in acute bronchitis
- worsening advice

References

Shadkam MN, Mozaffari-Khosravi H, Mozayan MR. A comparison of the effect of honey, dextromethorphan, and diphenhydramine on nightly cough and sleep quality in children and their parents. *J Altern Complement Med.* 2010; **16**(7): 787–93.

Timmer A, Günther J, Rücker G, *et al.* Pelargonium sidoides extract for acute respiratory tract infections. *Cochrane Database Syst Rev.* 2008; **3**: CD006323.

Specific treatment for acute cough will depend on the cause:

1 Acute bronchitis
2 Laryngitis
3 Pneumonia
4 COPD exacerbation
5 Asthma exacerbation
6 Viral-induced wheeze
7 Croup in children
8 Bronchiolitis in babies
9 Whooping cough in children

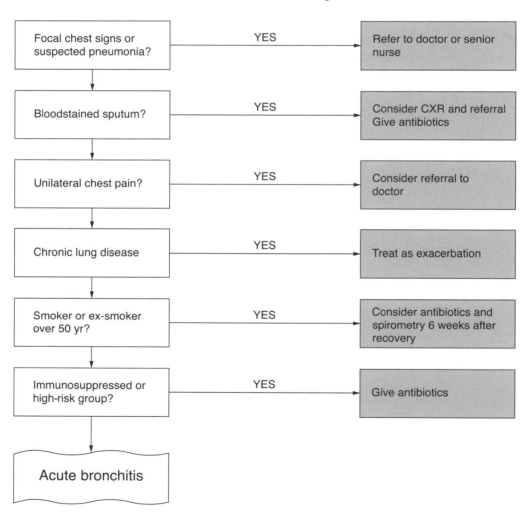

FIGURE 2.1 Adult with acute cough.

1. Acute bronchitis

- a viral or bacterial infection of adults or children
- fever
- cough (may be productive)
- maybe wheeze
- maybe central chest pain on coughing
- no other chest signs
- normal respiratory rate, pulse and BP

Antibiotics for acute bronchitis

Prescribe an antibiotic if:
- seriously ill
- high-risk group (*see* page 6)
- bloodstained sputum

Consider an antibiotic if:
- smoker over 50 (likely to have undiagnosed COPD – consider chest X-ray (CXR) now, and then spirometry 6 weeks after recovery from acute infection)
- prolonged or worsening symptoms

Antibiotic choice
- amoxicillin for 5 days (500 mg three times daily in adults)
- if allergic to penicillin, give clarithromycin
- if not responding to amoxicillin, add clarithromycin

Refer to doctor
- routinely if persistent or recurrent symptoms

References

Braman SS. Chronic cough due to acute bronchitis: ACCP evidence-based clinical practice guidelines. *Chest.* 2006; **129**(Suppl. 1): 95S–103S.

Cornford CS, Morgan M, Ridsdale L. Why do mothers consult when their children cough? *Fam Pract.* 1993; **10**: 193–6.

Johnson G, Helman C. Remedy or cure? Lay beliefs about over-the-counter medicines for coughs and colds. *BJGP.* 2004; **54**: 98–102.

Morice AH. *Cough.* Hull: International Society for the Study of Cough; 2007. Available at: www. issc.info

Prodigy. *Clinical topic: Chest infections – adult.* 2011. Available at: http://prodigy.clarity.co.uk/chest_infections_adult (accessed 29 August 2011).

Smith SM, Fahey T, Smucny J, *et al.* Antibiotics for acute bronchitis. *Cochrane Database Syst Rev.* 2004; **4**: CD000245.

Usmani OS, Belvisi MG, Patel HJ, *et al*. Theobromine inhibits sensory nerve activation and cough. *FASEB J*. 2005; **19**: 231–3.

2. Laryngitis

- a viral infection of adults and children
- symptoms: hoarseness, sore throat (worse on swallowing), fever, headache, dry irritating cough

Examination

- usually normal apart from fever

Self-care

- avoid smoky environments
- drink adequate fluids
- try not to swallow or cough more than essential
- take paracetamol or ibuprofen for headache
- rest your voice

Refer to doctor

- if hoarseness persists for more than 4 weeks (for Ear, Nose and Throat department referral)

3. Pneumonia

- an infection of the lung parenchyma, usually bacterial
- high mortality
- focal chest signs (e.g. dullness on percussion, bronchial breathing, coarse crackles)
- elderly people may have non-specific symptoms, and are less likely to have fever

History

- fever
- rigors
- cough
- breathlessness
- bloodstained or rusty sputum
- unilateral chest pain
- muscle or joint pain

Examination

- temperature
- rapid respiration
- tachycardia
- focal chest signs (e.g. dullness on percussion, bronchial breathing, coarse crackles)
- maybe low BP, prolonged CRT, low oxygen saturations

Test

- if smoker over 50, CXR now, and then spirometry 6 weeks after recovery
- if pneumonia confirmed, repeat CXR will be advised after 6 weeks

Action

- always give antibiotics
- review in 2–7 days

Antibiotic choice

- amoxicillin for 7 days (500 mg–1 g three times daily in adults)
- if allergic to penicillin, clarithromycin
- in more severe pneumonia, amoxicillin plus clarithromycin
- if following flu-like illness, treat for 14–21 days. Give co-amoxiclav (not amoxicillin, which does not cover staphylococcus). If patient is allergic to penicillin, give doxycycline in adults and clarithromycin in children
- if not responding to amoxicillin, add clarithromycin

 Refer to doctor

- urgently for possible hospital admission if:
    — severe illness
    — mental confusion
    — HIV infection (possible *Pneumocystis carinii* pneumonia)
    — breathless
    — unilateral chest pain, worse on coughing or deep breathing (suggests pleurisy, pulmonary embolism or pneumothorax)
    — recession
    — respiratory rate above 50/min under 1 year, 40/min under 6, 30/min or more age 6–adult
    — systolic BP of 90 mmHg or less or diastolic of 60 mmHg or less in adults
    — oxygen saturation below 95%
    — baby with abnormal chest examination (may be bronchiolitis, *see* page 22)

Caution

- pneumonia is not a minor illness, and should only be managed by experienced clinicians

References

Blackburn R, Henderson K, Lillie M, *et al*. Empirical treatment of influenza-associated pneumonia in primary care: a descriptive study of the antimicrobial susceptibility of lower respiratory tract bacteria (England, Wales and Northern Ireland, January 2007–March 2010). *Thorax*. 2011; doi: 10.1136/thx.2010.134643.

British Thoracic Society. *BTS Guidelines for the Management of Community Acquired Pneumonia in Adults*. London: British Thoracic Society; 2001. Available at: www.brit-thoracic.org.uk

4. COPD/bronchiectasis exacerbation

History

- sputum quantity
- sputum colour
- breathlessness
- fever
- recent antibiotics

Examination

- confusion
- cyanosis
- ankle oedema
- respiratory rate/distress
- oxygen saturation

Self-care

- increase dose or frequency of short-acting bronchodilator to the maximum (salbutamol or ipratropium)
- use spacer
- worsening advice

Prescription

- if breathlessness has worsened, give prednisolone 30 mg/day for 14 days

Antibiotics for COPD/bronchiectasis exacerbations

Prescribe an antibiotic:
- if sputum has become purulent (green and thick)

Antibiotic choice

- amoxicillin for 7 days (500 mg three times daily in adults)
- if allergic to penicillin, give clarithromycin
- if severe COPD with recurrent antibiotic use, consider doxycycline or co-amoxiclav
- if not responding to amoxicillin, add clarithromycin or change to doxycycline

Refer to doctor

- urgently if:
  - severe symptoms
  - increasing oedema
  - oxygen saturation < 95%

5. Asthma exacerbation

History

- cough
- wheeze
- breathlessness
- sleep disturbance
- fever
- previous hospital admissions for asthma
- current medication

Examination

- ability to complete sentence
- cyanosis
- respiratory rate
- pulse and blood pressure, in severe episodes
- peak flow
- oxygen saturation

Self-care

- immediately use salbutamol inhaler with a large-volume spacer:
  — give one puff at a time and inhale with five tidal breaths
    – adult: 4 puffs initially, followed by 2 puffs every 2 minutes according to response, up to 10 puffs
    – child: 2 puffs every 2 minutes according to response, up to 10 puffs
  — repeat every 10–20 minutes according to response
- use nebuliser if unable to manage spacer. Consider driving this with oxygen
- afterwards:
  — use inhaled salbutamol as required, up to four times a day (not more frequently than every 4 h)
  — do not increase the dose of inhaled steroid
  — worsening advice – monitor PEF and symptoms. If symptoms worsen or PEF decreases, seek further advice

Prescription

- do not give antibiotics
- give a short course of oral prednisolone:
  — child < 2 years: 10 mg daily for 3 days
  — child 2–5 years: 20 mg daily for 3 days
  — child 6–12 years: 30–40 mg daily for 3 days
  — adult or child > 12 years: 40–50 mg daily for 5 days

Refer to doctor or asthma specialist nurse
- urgently if:
  - — oxygen saturation < 95%
  - — exhaustion, inability to complete sentence
  - — brittle asthma with previous hospital admissions
  - — not responding to treatment
- routinely for follow up within 1 week

6. Viral-induced wheeze

Viral infections may cause wheezing and tightness in the chest in those who do not have asthma. Use salbutamol metered dose inhaler (MDI) via spacer, four times daily for 1 week. In children, those with a family history of atopy *and* exercise-induced wheeze are more likely to develop asthma later.

Refer to doctor or asthma specialist nurse
- routinely if not improving, or still needing bronchodilator after 1 week

Differential diagnosis of acute cough in children

As well as the conditions mentioned above, there are certain illnesses which may cause acute cough in children: bronchiolitis, croup and whooping cough.

TABLE 2.1 Differential diagnosis of acute cough with chest signs in children

	Pneumonia	Bronchiolitis	Viral-induced wheeze
Age	Any age	Under 1 year	12 months–5 years
Fever	Yes	Yes	Maybe
Respiratory rate	Increased	Increased	Normal or increased
Recession	No	Maybe	Maybe
Hyperinflation	No	Often	Maybe
Wheeze	No*	Maybe	Present
Crackles	Coarse, localised	Fine, generalised	No

* except with mycoplasma pneumonia
Adapted from Prodigy, *Clinical topic: Cough – acute with chest signs in children*

7. Bronchiolitis

- a viral infection of children under 12 months of age
- mainly caused by respiratory syncytial virus
- features: raised respiratory rate, fine generalized crackles and sometimes wheezes in chest, usually fever

Self-care

- maintain adequate fluid intake
- worsening advice:
  - faster breathing > 50/min
  - increasing difficulty in breathing
  - recession
  - reduced feeding (less than 50% of normal)
  - signs of dehydration
  - worsening fever

Refer to doctor

- urgently always (may be difficult to distinguish from pneumonia)

References

Prodigy. *Clinical topic: Cough – acute with chest signs in children*. 2011. Available at: <u>http://prodigy.clarity.co.uk/cough_acute_with_chest_signs_in_children</u> (accessed 29 August 2011).

Scottish Intercollegiate Guidelines Network (SIGN). *Bronchiolitis in Children: SIGN guideline 91*. Edinburgh: Scottish Intercollegiate Guidelines Network; 2006. <u>www.sign.ac.uk/pdf/sign91.pdf</u>

Umoren R, Odey F, Meremikwu MM. Steam inhalation or humidified oxygen for acute bronchiolitis in children up to three years of age. *Cochrane Database Syst Rev*. 2011; **1**: CD006435.

8. Croup

A viral infection of children aged between 3 months and 5 years.

History

- cough (often 'brassy' or 'barking')
- crowing noise on inspiration (stridor, worse at night)
- may be breathless

Examination

- temperature
- respiratory rate
- chest (usually normal)
- throat

Self-care

- explain nature of illness
- steam inhalations are often used, but their effectiveness is not proven. If the parent chooses to use them, advise placing bowl of hot water in basin or sink to reduce risk of scalds
- worsening advice

Prescription

- give all children with croup two doses of oral prednisolone (1–2 mg per kg body weight) 24 h apart. If it is impractical to weigh the child, give 10 mg prednisolone to children aged 6 months to 2 years

Refer to doctor

- urgently if:
  - immunosuppressed
  - recession
  - respiratory distress
  - parents not coping

References

Alberta Medical Association. *Guideline for the Diagnosis and Management of Croup*. Edmonton: Alberta Medical Association; 2008. Available at: www.topalbertadoctors.org

Russell K, Wiebe N, Saenz A, *et al*. Glucocorticoids for croup. *Cochrane Database Syst Rev.* 2004; **1**: CD001955.

Sparrow A, Geelhoed G. Prednisolone versus dexamethasone in croup: a randomised equivalence trial. *Arch Dis Child*. 2006; **91**(7): 580–3.

9. Whooping cough

- mainly affects babies and young children
- consider in child if coughing > 2 weeks
- especially if vomiting occurs after coughing
- even if they are fully immunised
- median duration of cough: 112 days
- examination of chest is usually normal
- notifiable disease

Tests

- < 2-week history: nasopharyngeal aspirate or nasal swab
- > 2-week history: serology

Antibiotic choice

- clarithromycin: reduces transmission, but does not benefit the patient

Reference

Hamder A, Grant C, Harrison T, *et al*. Whooping cough in school age children with persistent cough: prospective cohort study in primary care. *BMJ*. 2006: **333**: 174–7.

3

Ear, nose and throat

Sore throat

History
- patient's agenda – often pain relief
- duration
- history of fever
- rash
- heart valve problems
- medication already tried
- medication which may affect the bone marrow (agranulocytosis), e.g. immunosuppressants including corticosteroids, carbimazole, mirtazapine, sulfasalazine, clozapine, disease-modifying anti-rheumatic drugs (DMARDs)

Examination
- temperature (take into account any recent antipyretic)
- examine throat – asking the patient to yawn, take a deep breath or pant may improve the view. Consider using tongue depressor if back of throat not visible (but exclude epiglottitis first, *see* page 28). Assess inflammation of pharynx and look for exudates on tonsils
- check neck for enlarged lymph nodes (cervical lymphadenopathy)
- look for the macular rash of scarlet fever (small red patches, not raised)

Test
- urgent FBC should be requested if on medication potentially toxic to bone marrow. The safe course of action is to stop the potentially toxic drug until the FBC result is confirmed to be normal

Differential diagnosis
- sore throat
- glandular fever
- quinsy

- epiglottitis
- scarlet fever (*see* page 71)

Self-care

- most sore throats are viral and recover within 7 days
- paracetamol or ibuprofen will relieve pain
- saltwater mouthwash (half a teaspoon of salt in 250 mL water)
- cold drinks and ice cream may be soothing
- benzydamine mouthwash or spray, e.g. Difflam, available over the counter (OTC), may relieve the discomfort
- worsening advice: seek help if they develop difficulty in breathing or are unable to swallow enough fluids

Antibiotics

Antibiotics are of marginal benefit in sore throat, and at best will only shorten the illness by 16 hours. Against this must be weighed the cost to the patient (prescription charge, burden of medicine-taking, risk of side-effects) and to society (antibiotic resistance, medicalisation of illness).

Antibiotics for sore throat

Prescribe an antibiotic if:
- seriously ill
- prolonged and worsening symptoms
- immunosuppressed
- heart valve disease (risk of endocarditis)

Notes on the Centor criteria

NICE guideline CG69 recommended that antibiotics were considered for patients with three or more Centor criteria. These criteria were developed in 1981 in an attempt to identify patients with sore throat who had bacterial as opposed to viral infection, and comprise tonsillar exudate, tender anterior cervical lymphadenopathy, history of fever and an absence of cough. However, it has been shown that even if all four criteria are met, there is only a 50% chance that the infection is bacterial, and although there was a little more benefit from antibiotics in these patients, the number needed to treat (NNT) was 60. Therefore, we do not recommend routine use of the criteria.

Antibiotic choice

- phenoxymethylpenicillin (penicillin V) for 10 days
- if allergic to penicillin, use clarithromycin
- for children who are unable to swallow tablets, amoxicillin suspension may be used

instead. It tastes much better than phenoxymethylpenicillin suspension, and concordance is likely to be better because it is given three times daily

- if not responding to antibiotic, reassess and take throat swab. If further antibiotics are necessary, use metronidazole

 Refer to doctor

- urgently if:
  - — very sick, drooling, cannot swallow (possible *epiglottitis*, do not examine throat)
  - — large swelling around one tonsil (possible *quinsy*, may need surgery)
  - — taking medication which may be toxic to bone marrow. If this is suspected, take immediate advice from a doctor regarding stopping the medication

References

Spinks AB, Glasziou PP, Del Mar CB. Antibiotics for sore throat. *Cochrane Database Syst Rev.* 2006; 4: CD000023.

National Institute for Health and Clinical Excellence. *Respiratory Tract Infections: antibiotic prescribing. Prescribing of antibiotics for self-limiting respiratory tract infections in adults and children in primary care. NICE guideline 47.* London: NIHCE; 2008. www.nice.org.uk/guidance/CG69

Van Driel ML, De Sutter A, Deveugele M, *et al.* Are sore throat patients who hope for antibiotics actually asking for pain relief? *Ann Fam Med.* 2006; 4(6): 494–9.

Wethington JF. Double-blind study of benzydamine hydrochloride, a new treatment for sore throat. *Clin Ther.* 1985; 7(5): 641–6.

Specific types of sore throat

1 Glandular fever
2 Quinsy
3 Epiglottitis

1. Glandular fever

- age 15–25 most commonly affected
- often asymptomatic
- caused by Epstein-Barr virus
- long incubation period (1–2 months)
- transmission by saliva

Common symptoms

- fever
- sore throat
- malaise
- prolonged fatigue

Examination
- oedema of the uvula, or around the eyes
- petechial rash on the palate
- generalised lymphadenopathy
- maculopapular rash (both flat and raised red areas)
- jaundice
- enlargement of spleen

Test
- Paul-Bunnell or monospot blood test, after at least 7 days (slow to turn positive, and high false negative rate)

Cautions
- rupture of spleen, respiratory obstruction from large tonsils
- avoid strenuous activity for 3 weeks and contact sports (e.g. rugby) for 8 weeks
- avoid amoxicillin and ampicillin, which may cause a rash (the rash is disease-specific, not due to an allergy)

2. Quinsy (peritonsillar abscess)
- severe illness with high fever
- 'hot potato' voice
- trismus (unable to open mouth)
- deviated uvula
- *refer same day* to Ear, Nose and Throat (ENT)

3. Epiglottitis
- adults or children
- high fever
- severe sore throat
- difficulty and pain when swallowing
- respiratory distress, high-pitched sounds
- cyanosis
- muffled voice
- drooling
- do not attempt to examine throat
- *refer to ENT (blue-light emergency)*

Mouth

1 oral candidiasis
2 aphthous ulcers
3 herpes simplex stomatitis
4 hand, foot and mouth disease
5 dental infections

1. Oral candidiasis (thrush)

A fungal infection, common in babies, those using inhaled corticosteroids and the immunosuppressed.

History
- soreness
- difficulty in eating/drinking
- immunosuppressed

Examination
- white patches on tongue and oral mucosa that cannot easily be removed
- redness of tongue or denture contact areas
- cracked area at angle of lip (angular cheilitis)

Tests
- swabs are unhelpful because many healthy people carry candida in their mouth
- in adults, consider FBC, fasting blood glucose (FBG), HIV serology, folate and vitamin B_{12}

Self-care
- avoid reinfection from teats/nipples/dummies in babies
- good dental hygiene in adults
- for those using inhaled steroids, recommend using spacer (e.g. Aerochamber) and afterwards rinse mouth out with water
- miconazole oral gel (OTC over age of 4 months) is the most effective treatment

Prescription
- miconazole oral gel is recommended by Prodigy as first-line for all patients. In babies, parents should be advised to take care that the gel does not obstruct the throat; avoid application to the back of the throat and subdivide doses. A prescription will be required for babies under 4 months (unlicensed indication)
- nystatin suspension is an alternative, but not licensed under 1 month
- oral fluconazole 50–100 mg daily for 7 days may be used in severe or resistant cases in adults

References

Ainsworth S, Jones W. It sticks in our throats too. *BMJ*. 2009; **338**: a3178.

Prodigy. *Clinical topic: Candida – oral*. 2011. Available at: http://prodigy.clarity.co.uk/candida_oral (accessed 29 August 2011).

2. Aphthous ulcers

History

- painful ulcers
- may occur anywhere in the mouth, most commonly on the buccal mucosa (lining of the cheek)

Examination

- red, round lesions, sometimes with white crater

Self-care

- reduce oral trauma (e.g. softer toothbrush)
- chlorhexidine oral spray
- benzydamine spray

Prescription

- hydrocortisone muco-adhesive buccal tablets

Refer to doctor

- urgently if:
  - — persisting/enlarging ulcer (may be a carcinoma)
  - — ulceration affects other parts of body

Reference

Prodigy. *Clinical topic: Aphthous ulcer*. 2011. Available at: http://prodigy.clarity.co.uk/aphthous_ulcer (accessed 29 August 2011).

3. Hand, foot and mouth disease

See page 70.

4. Herpes simplex stomatitis

As well as the familiar cold sore (*see* page 72) the herpes simplex virus (HSV-1) when it is first encountered may cause a systemic illness with extensive mouth ulceration.

History
- usually a child under five
- short history of fever and malaise
- refusing to eat or drink

Examination
- temperature
- check for dehydration
- multiple small ulcers on tongue, palate and buccal mucosa (cheek lining)

Self-care
- ensure adequate fluid intake (a straw, or very cold drinks may help)
- use paracetamol (not ibuprofen) for pain relief
- benzydamine spray may be helpful
- apply Vaseline to lips
- take precautions to reduce infection spread
- avoid contact with babies aged under 4 weeks

Refer to doctor
- urgently if immunosuppressed, for consideration of oral aciclovir

Reference

Prodigy. *Clinical topic: Herpes simplex – oral.* 2011. Available at: http://prodigy.clarity.co.uk/herpes_simplex_oral (accessed 29 August 2011).

5. Dental infections

History
- pain, sudden onset and rapidly worsening, may radiate to ear or jaw
- bad taste in mouth
- fever and malaise
- when dentist last consulted
- previous treatment

Examination
- site of pain
- swelling
- dental decay

Self-care
- advise seeing dentist as soon as possible
- ibuprofen or naproxen, if tolerated, are the most effective analgesics
- paracetamol can be added
- the effect of codeine on dental pain is small

Prescription

- Give antibiotics if:
  — severe infection (e.g. fever, lymphadenopathy, cellulitis)
  — immunosuppressed
  — diabetes
  — heart valve disease
- high-dose, short-course amoxicillin
- metronidazole for 5 days if allergic to penicillin

References

Hargreaves K, Abbott PV. Drugs for pain management in dentistry. *Aust Dent J.* 2005; 50(4 Suppl. 2): S14–22.

Prodigy. *Clinical topic: Dental abscess.* 2011. Available at: http://prodigy.clarity.co.uk/dental_abscess (accessed 29 August 2011).

'Swollen glands' (enlarged cervical lymph nodes)

History

- sore throat
- fever
- duration of swelling

Examination

- number, location and size of enlarged nodes
- throat

Test

- if symptoms last more than a week:
  — FBC, erythrocyte sedimentation rate (ESR)
  — Paul-Bunnell/monospot if aged 15–25
  — consider HIV serology

Self-care

- explain that the 'glands' are the body's defence against infection
- take ibuprofen or paracetamol if pain is severe
- worsening advice: seek help if not settling after 3 weeks

Refer to doctor

- urgently if there is a single very large painful node (may contain an abscess)
- urgently if lymph nodes are hard or enlarging progressively over several weeks (may be a sign of HIV, lymphoma, leukaemia, sarcoidosis or tuberculosis)

Mumps

A viral infection of the salivary glands. This was previously a disease of children, which had become rare following the introduction of mumps vaccination. Most cases are without serious consequence, but complications include orchitis, pancreatitis, viral meningitis and risk of miscarriage between 12 and 16 weeks' gestation. In 2004, as a consequence of the mumps, measles and rubella (MMR) vaccine scare, there was a large increase in mumps cases in the 16–25 age group.

History
- swelling/pain of parotid glands
- dry mouth, worse on swallowing or chewing
- fever
- malaise
- headache
- earache
- drowsiness/photophobia/vomiting
- abdominal or testicular pain
- contact with mumps (up to 28 days before)

Examination
- parotid glands (swelling may be unilateral or bilateral)
- earlobe may be pushed aside

Tests
- confirmation of the diagnosis (using a special salivary sample kit) may be requested by the Health Protection Agency after the disease has been notified

Self-care
- paracetamol or ibuprofen may ease the discomfort
- maintain fluid intake
- acidic fruit juices may intensify the pain and should be avoided
- infectious for 5 days after the onset of swelling
- vulnerable contacts (who have not previously received two doses of mumps vaccine) should be vaccinated. Unfortunately, though, vaccination will not protect against infection this time
- worsening advice: seek help if severe headache, vomiting, neck stiffness, abdominal or testicular pain

Refer to doctor
- urgently if symptoms of meningitis, abdominal or testicular pain

Ear problems

History
- duration and type of pain/discomfort
- fever
- deafness
- discharge
- recent swimming or diving
- previous episodes (how treated and what happened)
- high-risk group

Examination
- temperature
- view ear from behind to look for outward and downward displacement (due to mastoiditis)
- check mastoid area for tenderness and swelling
- ear canal for inflammation, foreign body, discharge or swelling (generalised or local, e.g. boil)
- tympanic membrane, to assess colour, dullness, perforation, bulging/retracted, fluid level

Differential diagnosis
- the most likely causes of acute earache are otitis media, otitis externa, boil in the ear canal, or Eustachian tube dysfunction

Reference

Van den Aardweg MT, Rovers MM, de Ru JA, *et al.* A systematic review of diagnostic criteria for acute mastoiditis in children. *Otol Neurotol.* 2008; **29**(6): 751.

Otitis media

Otitis media is commonest in small children, though it may occur in adults. It causes pain, deafness and sometimes fever, vomiting and loss of balance. The eardrum is red. It may be bulging or a discharge may be present. If the history is suggestive but the drum cannot be seen (e.g. because of wax), it is safest to assume that otitis media is present. Pink eardrums are to be expected if other membranes are inflamed (e.g. conjunctivitis, red throat), or after crying.

Self-care
- recommend ibuprofen or paracetamol in maximum dosage
- explain that antibiotics are not helpful for the majority of patients with otitis media. Sixty per cent of patients will be pain-free within 24 h, whether or not they take antibiotics, and the chances of experiencing a side-effect from the antibiotic are greater than the chances of benefiting
- flying or diving may cause severe pain and perforation, and should be avoided while pain is present

- severe infections may cause temporary deafness by perforation of the eardrum, which will usually heal in 2 weeks
- reassure that ear infections very rarely cause permanent hearing damage

Antibiotics for otitis media

Prescribe an antibiotic if:
- seriously ill
- prolonged and worsening symptoms > 4 days
- immunosuppressed

Consider an antibiotic if:
- child younger than 2 years with bilateral otitis media
- child with perforation and discharge

NB: there is little evidence on the role of antibiotics in adults with otitis media.

Antibiotic choice
- amoxicillin 40 mg/kg/day in divided doses, i.e. 13.3 mg/kg three times a day (up to a maximum of 1 g three times a day) for 5 days
- if allergic to penicillin, give clarithromycin
- if not responding to amoxicillin, change to co-amoxiclav

Refer to doctor
- urgently if suspected mastoiditis (ENT referral)
- routinely if hearing does not return to normal within 14 days, for monitoring of perforation

References
Sanders S, Glasziou PP, Del Mar CB, *et al*. Antibiotics for acute otitis media in children. *Cochrane Database Syst Rev*. 1999; **3**: CD000219.

Scottish Intercollegiate Guidelines Network (SIGN). *Diagnosis and Management of Childhood Otitis Media in Primary Care: SIGN guideline 66*. Edinburgh: Scottish Intercollegiate Guidelines Network; 2003. www.sign.ac.uk/pdf/sign66.pdf

Otitis externa

This is a form of infected eczema which causes itchy discomfort rather than pain. It may follow inappropriate probing of the ear with a hairgrip or cotton bud, or the presence of a foreign body. It may be recurrent. Insertion of the auriscope is often uncomfortable. The canal looks irregular, red or moist, perhaps with discharge. Fungal infection may be present, especially after the use of antibiotic drops.

Test
- consider taking a swab if there is copious discharge, resistant or recurrent infection

Self-care
- avoid putting anything into the ear canal
- use cotton wool and Vaseline to keep shampoo and shower gel out of inflamed ears while showering or washing hair
- dry inside ears with hairdryer on lowest setting
- use earplugs when swimming; avoid swimming while ear is inflamed
- use acetic acid spray (Earcalm, OTC) before swimming, after swimming, at bedtime and at the first sign of irritation

Prescription
- if very inflamed, offer Otosporin eardrops for 7 days. Locorten-Vioform is an alternative but Otosporin is preferable after swimming, hot tubs, or with vivid green exudate from the ear, as pseudomonas may be responsible
- if unable to use eardrops, Otomize spray

Antibiotics for otitis externa

Prescribe an oral antibiotic if:
- signs of systemic infection
- cellulitis
- canal completely blocked with debris
- immunosuppressed
- diabetes

Antibiotic choice
- flucloxacillin for 7 days
- if patient is allergic to penicillin, give clarithromycin
- if swab shows pseudomonas and topical treatment ineffective, may need ciprofloxacin

Refer to doctor

- urgently if severe infection in high-risk patient with diabetes or immunosuppression ('malignant' otitis externa extending into bone)
- routinely if persistent/recurrent symptoms, for consideration of ENT referral for microsuction

References

Osguthorpe JD, Nielsen DR. Otitis externa: review and clinical update. *Am Fam Physician*. 2006; **74**(9): 1510–16.

Kaushik V, Malik T, Saeed SR. Interventions for acute otitis externa. *Cochrane Database Syst Rev*. 2010; **1**: CD004740.

Boil in ear canal

This causes a localised red swelling in the canal, often with unilateral deafness and severe pain on insertion of the auriscope.

Self-care

- take paracetamol or ibuprofen to relieve the pain
- the ear may discharge

Antibiotics for boil in ear canal

Prescribe an antibiotic if:
- cellulitis spreading to pinna
- fever
- immunosuppressed
- diabetes

Antibiotic choice

- flucloxacillin for 7 days
- if patient is allergic to penicillin, give clarithromycin

Reference

Prodigy. *Clinical topic: Localised otitis externa*. 2011. Available at: http://prodigy.clarity.co.uk/otitis_externa/view_whole_topic#-293574 (accessed 29 August 2011).

Eustachian tube dysfunction

This may follow an episode of otitis media or upper respiratory tract infection (URTI). It is commoner in children. The hearing is impaired and the ear is intermittently uncomfortable. The eardrum may appear normal, retracted or bulging. A fluid level may be seen behind the drum, which is not inflamed.

Self-care
- explain that the eardrum is a sensitive structure that hurts when the pressure changes. When catarrh blocks the Eustachian tube, changes in atmospheric pressure cause earache that comes and goes
- nasal decongestants, e.g. ephedrine drops, for no more than 7 days
- try to 'pop' the ears
- paracetamol or ibuprofen will ease the discomfort
- menthol and eucalyptus inhalations may be tried for adults

Refer to doctor
- routinely if not improving after 2 weeks (may need ENT referral)

Ear wax

Wax is a mixture of several substances, including dead skin cells, cerumen (produced by special glands in the ear canal) and sebum from sebaceous glands. It is mildly acidic and antibacterial. Jaw movement causes it to travel towards the outside of the ear, so it cleans and lubricates the ear canal.

History
- deafness
- ear discomfort/blockage
- tinnitus
- itching
- use of cotton buds

Examination
- note extent of wax and whether it is impacted against tympanic membrane

Self-care
- do not insert cotton buds inside the ear canal
- use olive oil ear drops, at body temperature, three times daily for 5 days
- the use of ear candles is not supported by evidence

Action
- if self-care is ineffective, consider irrigation (syringing). Contraindications to irrigation include:
  — perforation of the tympanic membrane. Some ENT specialists may permit irrigation if there is an old healed perforation, but this should be agreed upon in advance
  — grommets
  — previous ear surgery
  — discharge from ear in the previous 12 months
  — otitis media in the previous 6 weeks
  — cleft palate, even after surgical correction
  — current otitis externa
  — foreign body in the ear
  — previous problem with irrigation

Reference

Prodigy. *Clinical topic: Ear wax*. 2011. Available at: http://prodigy.clarity.co.uk/earwax/evidence/references#-286395 (accessed 29 August 2011).

Common cold (coryza or URTI)

History
- duration
- sore throat
- hoarse voice
- productive cough
- joint and muscle pains
- fever

Examination
- throat (usually appears normal)
- cervical lymph nodes
- ears
- chest

Self-care
- paracetamol or ibuprofen for sore throat and headache
- steam or menthol inhalations or menthol rubs for nasal congestion
- gargling with saltwater (half a teaspoon of salt in 250 mL water)
- sodium chloride nasal drops (for babies) or spray (e.g. Stérimar Hypertonic)
- chlorphenamine at night may help congestion and aid sleep
- nasal decongestant drops or sprays, e.g. ephedrine, for no more than 7 days

- some evidence suggests that high-dose zinc and vitamin C, echinacea and pelargonium preparations (e.g. Kaloba) may shorten the duration of colds

References

Arroll B. Non-antibiotic treatments for upper-respiratory tract infections (common cold). *Resp Med*. 2005; **99**(12): 1477–84.

Hemilä H. Zinc Lozenges may shorten the duration of colds: a systematic review. *Open Resp Med J*. 2011; **5**: 51–8.

Hemilä H, Chalker E, Douglas B. Vitamin C for preventing and treating the common cold. *Cochrane Database Syst Rev*. 2007; **3**: CD000980.

Linde K, Barrett B, Wolkart K, *et al*. Echinacea for preventing and treating the common cold. *Cochrane Database Syst Rev*. 2006; **1**: CD000530.

Singh M, Das RR. Zinc for the common cold. *Cochrane Database Syst Rev*. 2011; **2**: CD001364.

Timmer A, Günther J, Rücker G, *et al*. Pelargonium sidoides extract for acute respiratory tract infections. *Cochrane Database Syst Rev*. 2008; **3**: CD006323.

Sinusitis

This condition is very difficult to diagnose because the traditional symptoms and signs are unreliable.

History
- duration – average 18–20 days
- nasal blockage
- purulent nasal discharge
- facial pain
- visual disturbance
- fever
- previous episodes: how treated
- high-risk group

Examination
- there are no reliable signs of sinusitis, but check:
  — temperature
  — throat (post-nasal discharge)
  — ears
  — localised swelling on forehead

Self-care
- irrigate the nose with sodium chloride solution (e.g. Stérimar Hypertonic)
- warm face packs
- avoid smoky atmospheres
- analgesia with paracetamol or ibuprofen
- ephedrine nasal drops (for no more than 7 days)

- most sinusitis is caused by viruses, and only one person in fifteen will benefit from antibiotics

Antibiotics for sinusitis

Prescribe an antibiotic if:
- seriously ill
- immunosuppressed
- prolonged and worsening symptoms > 7 days

Antibiotic choice
- amoxicillin 1 g three times daily for 7 days
- if allergic to penicillin, give doxycycline or clarithromycin
- if not responding, change to co-amoxiclav or azithromycin

Refer to doctor
- urgently if periorbital oedema, double vision, reduced visual acuity or swelling of the forehead (intraorbital or intracranial complications)
- urgently if second-line antibiotics ineffective
- routinely if more than three episodes of sinusitis requiring antibiotics in 1 year

References

Ahovuo-Saloranta A, Rautakorpi U-M, Borisenko OV, *et al*. Antibiotics for acute maxillary sinusitis. *Cochrane Database Syst Rev.* 2008; **2**: CD000243.

Harvey R, Hannan SA, Badia L, *et al*. Nasal saline irrigations for the symptoms of chronic rhinosinusitis. *Cochrane Database Syst Rev.* 2007; **3**: CD006394.

Hay fever

History
- seasonal (usually April to August)
- frequent sneezing
- blocked nose
- red, itchy, watery eyes
- dry, sore throat
- wheeze, chest tightness, cough
- has patient tried any over-the-counter treatment
- if so, with what effect

Examination
- check eyes for discharge (suggests infection)

Self-care

- avoid long grass, fragrant flowers and newly mowed lawns
- when choosing a car, consider a pollen filter
- there is no evidence to support the standard advice to sleep with windows closed
- saline nasal douching is helpful (*see* 'Stérimar Hypertonic', page 40)
- steroid nasal sprays (OTC) reduce nasal symptoms more than oral antihistamines, but have no proven effect on eye symptoms
- nasal decongestants such as ephedrine drops (OTC) relieve nasal blockage, but should not be used for more than 7 days
- oral antihistamines such as cetirizine (OTC) reduce all hay fever symptoms. Even 'non-drowsy' preparations may not be permitted for people in safety-critical occupations
- they are more effective if started a few days before symptoms are expected to begin
- there is no evidence that one antihistamine is better than others overall, but individual patients may differ in their response
- if a topical antihistamine is preferred, Otrivine Antistin eye drops for no more than 7 days (OTC)
- sodium cromoglicate eye drops can be bought OTC as an additional treatment, but are slow to take effect

TABLE 3.1 Recommended medication for hay fever

Hay fever medication	Over the counter	Prescription
Steroid nasal spray	Best value	Budesonide
Antihistamine – oral	Best value	Cetirizine
Antihistamine – eye	Otrivine Antistin (for no more than 7 days)	Azelastine
Long-term eye drops	Sodium cromoglicate	Sodium cromoglicate

Prescriptions

- nasal symptoms: regular budesonide nasal spray, started 1 week before the hay fever season starts. Alternatively, consider nasal azelastine if symptoms are infrequent, as it has a quicker onset and can be used 'as required'
- antihistamine: oral (cetirizine) or ocular (azelastine)
- mast cell stabilizer: sodium cromoglicate eye drops
- in severe cases, prednisolone 15–20 mg daily in adults (5–10 mg daily in children) for 7 days

Refer to doctor

- routinely if symptoms persist after various combinations of the above have been tried

References

Harvey R, Hannan SA, Badia L, *et al*. Nasal saline irrigations for the symptoms of chronic rhinosinusitis. *Cochrane Database Syst Rev*. 2007; **3**: CD006394.

Scadding GK, Durham SR, Mirakian R, *et al*. BSACI guidelines for the management of allergic and non-allergic rhinitis. *Clin Exp Allergy*. 2008; **38**(1): 19–42.

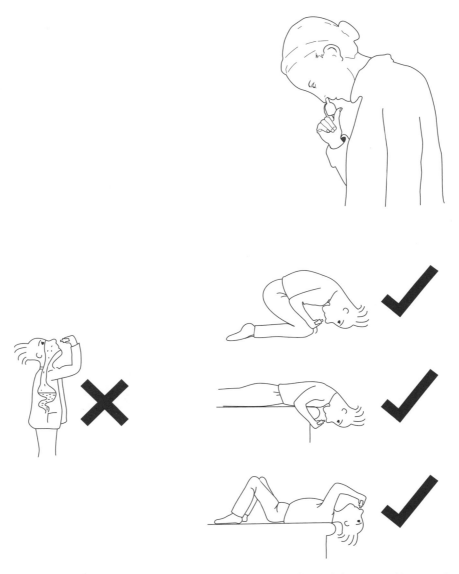

FIGURE 3.1 The correct use of nasal sprays (above) and drops (below) (from Scadding *et al.*, 2008).

To use a nasal spray:

- shake bottle well
- look down
- using *right* hand for *left* nostril, put nozzle just inside nose, aiming towards outside wall
- squirt once or twice (two different directions)
- change hands and repeat for other side
- *do not sniff hard*

4

Eyes

Sore eyes

History
- duration
- contacts (e.g. sibling)
- associated cold symptoms
- any problem with vision
- discharge
- diabetes
- previous eye problems, e.g. iritis
- history of trauma/foreign body/drilling or grinding, especially metal
- contact lens use

Examination
- in uncomplicated conjunctivitis, no examination may be necessary
- normal visual acuity is the most helpful sign in excluding a serious eye condition
- discharge
- redness
- bilateral or unilateral
- pupils equal and react to light
- look for foreign body (evert eyelid), especially if symptoms unilateral
- scales at roots of eyelashes (blepharitis)
- lids (stye, meibomian cyst, cellulitis)
- painful clusters of spots around eye (possible shingles)

Tests
- take bacterial and chlamydial swabs if persistent or recurrent symptoms. Remember that it is necessary to press firmly with a chlamydial swab
- stain with fluorescein if unilateral/history of trauma/recent use of power tools (but do not use with contact lens in situ)

Action
- depends on cause (see below)

Refer to doctor
- urgently if:
  — history of drilling or grinding, especially metal
  — severe inflammation
  — pain, not gritty discomfort
  — photophobia
  — reduced visual acuity
  — unequal/irregular pupils
  — any abnormality seen using fluorescein
  — previous serious eye disease
  — persistent/recurrent symptoms
  — baby under 4 weeks with red eye

Infective conjunctivitis

Sore eyes, red conjunctival membranes, usually with discharge. May be unilateral, especially in early stages. Check for scales on roots of eyelashes; if present, *see* 'Blepharitis' (page 48).

Self-care
- remove contact lenses, if worn, until problem has completely settled. Advise patient to see optometrist if symptoms are recurrent
- should settle without treatment in 1–2 weeks
- clean discharge away with cotton wool soaked in water
- lubricant eye drops such as Viscotears may reduce discomfort
- viral conjunctivitis is very likely if associated URTI
- chloramphenicol makes little difference to comfort or speed of recovery and should not be used unless symptoms are severe
- up to 10% of people treated with chloramphenicol suffer adverse reactions
- if used, chloramphenicol eyedrops should be applied as often as possible (every 3 h ideally initially). If severe, apply ointment at night also (treat only the infected eye(s))
- wash hands after touching eyes, use own facecloth, make-up, pillowcase and towel. If used, mascara and eyeliner may carry bacteria
- although the Health Protection Agency (HPA) does not recommend exclusion, schools and nurseries often prefer that children with conjunctivitis do not attend until discharge has cleared
- complications are rare, but urgently seek advice if:
  — severe eye pain or photophobia
  — visual problems
  — eye redness becomes severe

Action

- chloramphenicol is not available OTC for children aged under 2 years, so if it is indicated then a prescription should be issued. Ointment may be easier to apply in babies
- fusidic acid drops are an alternative which is narrower in spectrum, but if indicated should be prescribed if:
  — pregnant
  — history of blood dyscrasias, such as aplastic anaemia
  — chloramphenicol allergy
  — frequent application is impractical, e.g. a housebound woman with rheumatoid arthritis who lives alone

Refer to doctor

- see list above under 'sore eyes'

References

Health Protection Agency. *Guidance on Infection Control in Schools and Other Child Care Settings*. London: Health Protection Agency; 2006. Available at: www.hpa.org.uk

National Prescribing Centre. Most people with acute infective conjunctivitis don't need antibiotics – even when the cause is bacterial. *MeReC Rapid Review*. 17 October 2011. www.npc.nhs.uk/rapidreview/?p=4543 (accessed 15 November 2011).

Rietveld R, Van Weert CPM, Ter Riet G, *et al*. Diagnostic impact of signs and symptoms in acute infectious conjunctivitis: systematic literature search. *BMJ*. 2003; **327**: 789.

Sheikh A, Hurwitz B. Antibiotics versus placebo for acute bacterial conjunctivitis. *Cochrane Database Syst Rev*. 2006; **2**: CD001211.

Allergic conjunctivitis

- bilateral itchy eyes
- generalised conjunctival inflammation
- recurrent symptoms
- sneezing, itchy throat
- history of triggers, e.g. animal fur, hay fever
- watering rather than discharge

Self-care

- avoid triggers, if possible
- oral antihistamine (cetirizine)
- an antihistamine eye drop is available OTC (Otrivine Antistin), but this also contains a vasoconstrictor so should not be used for more than 7 days
- sodium cromoglicate eye drops are an alternative, but are slower acting

Action
- if self-care ineffective, prescribe azelastine eyedrops
- if patient pregnant or breastfeeding, prescribe sodium cromoglicate eyedrops

Reference
Owen CG, Shah A, Henshaw K, *et al*. Topical treatments for seasonal allergic conjunctivitis: systematic review and meta-analysis of efficacy and effectiveness. *Brit J Gen Pract*. 2004; 54(503): 451–6.

Dry eyes
Older patients more commonly affected, eyes feel gritty but look normal, vision unaffected.
- artificial tears help if used frequently (Viscotears OTC)
- omega-3 supplements may be useful

Reference
Wojtowicz JC, Butovich I, Uchiyama E, *et al*. Pilot, prospective, randomized, double-masked, placebo-controlled clinical trial of an omega-3 supplement for dry eye. *Cornea*. 2011; 30(3): 308–14.

Blepharitis
Conjunctivitis with infected scales at roots of eyelashes. There may be an associated seborrhoeic dermatitis.
- apply chloramphenicol eye ointment
- remove scales by applying warm compresses, then wiping lids twice daily for 2 weeks with cotton wool dipped in diluted baby shampoo, or a pinch of sodium bicarbonate in a cup of cooled, boiled water. Long-term lid hygiene should be recommended
- dry eyes often coexist – see above

Refer to doctor
- same day if:
  — abnormal shape or reaction of pupils to light
  — reduced visual acuity
  — foreign body in eye or under eyelid which you cannot remove with irrigation/moist cotton bud
  — persistent/recurrent symptoms
  — severe inflammation
  — shingles/herpes simplex suspected
  — any abnormality seen using fluorescein

Caution
- iritis (reduced visual acuity, unequal/irregular pupils, photophobia)
- chlamydia (pale bumps on inner lids – neonates are most commonly affected)

- herpes (cold sores, shingles)
- contact lens problems (consult optometrist)

Reference

American Academy of Ophthalmology. *Blepharitis*. San Francisco, CA: American Academy of
Ophthalmology; 2003. Available at: www.aao.org

Subconjunctival haemorrhage

This may sometimes be confused with conjunctivitis. It causes a sudden uniform red area in the eye with a sharp edge. You should be able to see the posterior margin. There is no discomfort, discharge or deterioration in vision. There is an association between this type of haemorrhage and high blood pressure or contact lens use. Also consider checking the INR if the patient is taking warfarin. Lubricant drops such as Viscotears may help to ease any discomfort.

Reference

Pitts JF, Jardine AG, Murray SB, Barker NH. Spontaneous subconjunctival haemorrhage – a sign
of hypertension? *Br J Ophthalmol*. 1992; **76**: 297–9.

Stye

- staphylococcal infection of the eyelash root
- on lash margin (swelling deeper in the lid would indicate a chalazion (meibomian cyst))
- any associated conjunctivitis or cellulitis

Self-care

- warm compresses 3–4 times daily
- consider pulling out eyelash or puncturing with sterile needle
- advise about infectiousness, use own facecloth and towel

Prescription

- if there is any sign of cellulitis of the eyelid, give antibiotics (*see* page 81)

Chalazion (meibomian cyst)

- caused by blockage in drainage of an eyelid gland
- swelling in eyelid, not on lash margin
- warm compresses 3–4 times daily to liquefy cyst contents
- massage cyst in direction of eyelash twice daily using clean fingers or cotton buds
- clean eyelid with cotton bud dipped in baby shampoo diluted 1 : 10 with warm water
- usually resolves without surgery in 6–8 weeks

Reference

Prodigy. *Clinical topic: Meibomian cyst*. 2011. Available at: http://prodigy.clarity.co.uk/meibomian_
cyst/evidence/references#-409170 (accessed 29 August 2011).

5

Head, neck and back

Headache

Only about 10% of headaches have a treatable cause. Less than 0.5% are serious. Severe headaches are not necessarily the ones of greater concern. Headache is a very common feature of many infections, but when infection has been ruled out the commonest cause of headache is stress.

History
- what is worrying you? (often a brain tumour)
- duration
- onset: sudden/gradual
- when: pain waking from sleep/later in the day/at night
- quality: sharp/like a pressure or band/throbbing
- site
- exacerbating factors, e.g. coughing, bending
- associated symptoms:
  - visual disturbance/eye pain
  - nausea
  - viral illness
  - sinus problems
  - neck pain
  - scalp or temple tenderness
  - neurological symptoms, e.g. sensory disturbance, double vision, incoordination
- previous recurrent headaches
- recent head injury
- previous cancer
- depression/anxiety/insomnia
- sleep pattern/shift work
- carbon monoxide exposure
- fluid, alcohol and caffeine intake
- oestrogen-containing contraceptives

- possibility of pregnancy
- treatment tried/effect/how long taken
- we all get headaches – what is different about this one?

Examination

- temperature
- blood pressure (this has to be really high – above 200/115 mmHg – to cause headache)
- palpate temporal arteries for tenderness, if over 50 years
- neck or back stiffness
- observe face for signs of swelling

Tests

- erythrocyte sedimentation rate (ESR) in patients aged over 50

TABLE 5.1 Features of a suspicious headache

Reassuring	Suspicious
On the top of my head	Always there when I wake up
Like a band around my head	Wakes me from sleep
It can last all day	Localised
It can come on at any time	Sudden onset
I've had it for years on and off	Hurts more when I cough or bend over
	Associated with neurological or visual symptoms

Self-care

- reassure (if appropriate) that headache without neurological or visual symptoms is very unlikely to indicate brain tumour
- regular meals, adequate fluids, avoid caffeine
- stress reduction or management (e.g. exercise, relaxation techniques)
- simple analgesics, e.g. ibuprofen (most people have only tried paracetamol)
- adequate, not excessive, time for sleep
- avoid codeine (increased risk of analgesic overuse headache)

Refer to doctor

- immediately if:
  — sudden 'thunderclap' headache (cerebral haemorrhage)
  — recent head injury (subdural haemorrhage)
  — suspicion of meningitis or carbon monoxide poisoning
  — eye pain (acute glaucoma)
  — headache waking from sleep (cerebral tumour, cluster headache)
  — neurological symptoms (cerebral haemorrhage/tumour)
  — temporal artery tenderness (giant cell arteritis)
  — pregnant and BP > 140/90

- routinely if:
  — simple analgesics taken for more than 15 days per month or opioids/triptans for more than 10 days per month ('medication-overuse headaches')
  — worsening/persistent headaches
  — underlying mental health problem

Note: there is no point in referring a patient presenting with headache and no eye symptoms to an optician. Poor vision is most unlikely to be the sole cause of headache, and if you are concerned enough to feel that the patient needs examination of the optic disc for signs of raised intracranial pressure, then urgent referral to a doctor is needed.

References

Bal SK, Hollingworth GR. 10-minute consultation: headache. *BMJ.* 2005; **330**: 346.

British Association for the Study of Headache. *Guidelines for All Healthcare Professionals in the Diagnosis and Management of Migraine, Tension-Type, Cluster and Medication-Overuse Headache.* Hull: British Association for the Study of Headache; 2007. Available at: www. bash.org.uk

Derry S, Moore RA, McQuay HJ. Paracetamol (acetaminophen) with or without an antiemetic for acute migraine headaches in adults. *Cochrane Database Syst Rev.* 2010; **11**: CD008040.

Scottish Intercollegiate Guidelines Network (SIGN). *Diagnosis and Management of Headache in Adults: SIGN guideline 107.* Edinburgh: Scottish Intercollegiate Guidelines Network; 2008. www.sign.ac.uk/pdf/sign107.pdf

---

Box 5.1 Giant cell (temporal) arteritis

This autoimmune condition causes inflammation in small to medium-sized arteries, especially those on the temples. It is more common over the age of 50 years, but may affect younger people. The headache is severe, often associated with tenderness of the scalp, aching of the jaw muscles on eating and visual disturbance. There may be associated weakness of other muscles with morning stiffness, aches and weight loss (polymyalgia rheumatica). It is a 'red flag' because it may cause sudden occlusion of important blood vessels, resulting in blindness, stroke or myocardial infarction, so patients in whom it is suspected should be referred urgently to a doctor. A raised ESR will help in confirming the diagnosis. Long-term treatment is needed with prednisolone 50 mg/day, aspirin 75 mg/day and omeprazole 20 mg/day.

Reference

Warrington KJ, Matteson EL. Management guidelines and outcome measures in giant cell arteritis (GCA). *Clin Exp Rheumatol.* 2007; **25**(6 Suppl. 47): 137–41.

Box 5.2 Migraine

Migraine affects 12% of adults and 10% of children, and is commoner in females. Symptoms of the aura do not last more than 60 minutes (typically 20–30 minutes), and resolve before the pain begins. Early symptoms, such as emotional or personality changes, muddled thinking, excessive tiredness, yawning, pallor, visual disturbances and restlessness, may start many hours before the headache. In children, visual symptoms are less common, but they may have abdominal pain, vomiting and dizziness.

Migraine is associated with abnormal changes in the size of the blood vessels in the head and neck, although the initial event that starts an attack occurs in the brainstem. It is helpful for patients to be informed that the reason they are susceptible to migraine, resulting from triggers that do not cause headache in other people, is an inherited predisposition.

A wide variety of factors are known to trigger migraine:
- change in stress level
- excessive sensory stimuli, e.g. bright light, noise
- menstruation
- long periods without eating
- overexertion
- sleep disturbance – too much or too little
- change in climate
- hypoxia

Dietary factors are often suspected but rarely found, and searching too hard may divert attention away from more likely factors such as those above. Alcohol does not cause migraine initially, but can trigger an attack when its effects wear off. For most people, the attacks seem to be multifactorial, and it is often not possible to identify any one trigger, which either always causes migraine or, when avoided, stops all attacks. Often there is a build-up of different triggers, with a 'last straw' tripping over the threshold, resulting in an attack. Whatever the cause, the final part of the sequence of events leading to symptoms involves the neurotransmitter 5-hydroxytryptamine (serotonin, 5-HT). Migraine associated with difficulty in reading, particularly in children or young people, may respond to colour tinting of spectacles. Referral to an optometrist for an intuitive colorimeter test may both help the migraine and (importantly) improve educational potential. Adults with frequent dyspepsia or heartburn as well as migraine should be referred to a doctor for investigation. If the presence of *Helicobacter pylori* is confirmed, eradication therapy may abolish the migraine as well as the gut symptoms.

History

- episodes lasting 4–72 h
- often unilateral (though not always)
- pulsating/throbbing
- moderate or severe pain
- worse after physical activity
- nausea and/or vomiting
- photophobia or phonophobia (sensitivity to noise)
- focal migraine will also cause one of the following types of aura:
  - visual symptoms (e.g. flickering lights and/or partial visual loss)
  - sensory symptoms (pins and needles and/or numbness)
  - dysphasia (speech disturbance)

Self-care

- patients often know a remedy that works for them, for example, a cup of tea, a lie-down in a quiet room and a short sleep
- when this is either impractical or ineffective, then drugs have a role
- simple analgesics (paracetamol, aspirin or ibuprofen) work for many people, but they must be taken early in the attack
- if there is associated nausea, it is important to treat this as well with an anti-emetic such as domperidone, ideally taken at the first sign of symptoms
- if simple analgesics are ineffective, consider sumatriptan (OTC)

Advice

- if taking combined oral contraceptive (COC) and first episode of migraine, or migraine with aura/focal symptoms, advise stopping COC immediately and discuss alternative methods

Refer to doctor

- urgently if migraine lasting more than 72 h
- routinely if:
  - simple analgesics and anti-emetics ineffective, to discuss triptans
  - frequent attacks (consider prophylaxis)

References

Gasbarrini A, De Luca A, Fiore G, *et al*. Beneficial effects of *Helicobacter pylori* eradication on migraine. *Hepato-Gastroenterol*. 1998; 45: 765–70.

Goadsby PJ. Recent advances in the diagnosis and management of migraine. *BMJ*. 2006; **332**: 25–9.

Machlachlan A, Yale S, Wilkins A. Open trial of subjective precision tinting: a follow-up of 55 patients. *Ophthalmic Physiol Optic*. 1993; **13**: 175–8.

<table>
<tr><td colspan="2">Box 5.3 Pre-eclampsia</td></tr>
</table>

- usually in the second half of first pregnancy
- first pregnancy with a new partner or in subsequent pregnancies after previous episodes
- severe increasing headaches
- visual problems, e.g. blurred vision, flashing lights, double vision
- pain or pain in epigastrium or right upper quadrant
- vomiting
- breathlessness
- swelling of face, hands, or feet
- may have proteinuria

Refer to doctor
- urgently if pregnant and BP > 140/90

Dizziness

History
- what is worrying you? (often a stroke)
- duration
- circumstances (during exercise or lying down suggests cardiac cause)
- nature ('when you have dizzy spells, do you feel light-headed or do you see the world spin around you as if you had just got off a playground roundabout?'):
  — spinning or movement (vertigo – *see* Box 5.4, page 57)
  — or faint feeling (as if about to black out)
- associated symptoms:
  — nausea
  — earache/deafness/tinnitus
  — headache/photophobia
  — palpitations
  — viral infection
- previous episodes
- recent head injury/blood loss
- pregnancy
- heart disease
- medication (e.g. antihypertensives)
- family history of sudden adult death
- if loss of consciousness, try to obtain written eyewitness account

Examination
- blood pressure sitting and standing
- pallor
- anaemia

Tests
- FBC if anaemia suspected
- electrocardiogram (ECG) if cardiac cause suspected

Self-care
- dizziness is common and often accompanies viral infections
- it will usually settle, but may sometimes take several weeks
- bed rest may be needed for a few days
- sit and stand slowly
- driving or other critical tasks may be affected

Refer to doctor
- urgently if:
  — neurological symptoms or signs
  — headache
  — recent head injury
  — heart disease, known or suspected
  — family history of sudden adult death
- routinely if:
  — on antihypertensive treatment and blood pressure low
  — persistent/recurrent symptoms
  — elderly

Box 5.4 Vertigo

In primary care, the commonest cause of acute vertigo is a viral infection (vestibular neuronitis). This infection was previously called labyrinthitis, but this term is now reserved for a more serious infection which also causes unilateral deafness. Acute vertigo may also represent the onset of a more long-term problem, such as benign paroxysmal positional vertigo or Menière's disease.

In patients with vertigo, examine the ears and check for nystagmus (a side-to-side eye movement, sometimes only seen on sideways gaze).

Self-care
- symptoms may take several weeks to resolve completely
- bed rest may be needed if symptoms are severe
- avoid driving, operating machinery
- consider prochlorperazine (buccal form available OTC, though only licensed for nausea) or cinnarizine (OTC)

Refer to doctor

- if sudden-onset deafness
- if previous ear surgery
- if not improving after 1 week
- if persisting after 6 weeks

Reference

Prodigy. *Clinical topic: Vertigo.* 2011. Available at: http://prodigy.clarity.co.uk/vertigo (accessed 29 August 2011).

Neck pain

History

- what is worrying you? (often meningitis)
- duration
- injury, e.g. whiplash
- neurological symptoms
- sore throat
- occupation (e.g. checkout/keyboard operator)
- change in sleeping position

Examination

- temperature (if infection suspected)
- cervical lymph nodes
- range of movement
- neck stiffness (can a child kiss his knees?)

Self-care

- reassure about meningitis (if appropriate)
- reassure that neck pain is common and likely to resolve in 3–4 weeks
- continue normal activity as much as possible
- sleep with one pillow
- try to maintain good posture
- consider workstation assessment
- do not drive if neck movements are restricted
- analgesia with ibuprofen/paracetamol
- if oral non-steroidal anti-inflammatory drug (NSAID) not possible and pain is muscular, consider a topical NSAID

Refer to doctor if:

- severe pain
- neurological symptoms

- rheumatoid arthritis
- localised tenderness over one vertebra

Back pain

History
- what is worrying you? (often prolonged debility)
- onset: gradual/sudden/while lifting
- duration/previous episodes
- site – make sure it really is in the back, not the kidney, lung or hip
- radiation to leg – especially below the knee
- numbness/tingling of leg
- difficulty passing urine/disturbed sensation in perineum
- fever
- abdominal pain/coldness/cyanosis of legs
- weight loss/malaise
- osteoporosis, known or risk
- previous cancer
- occupation
- psychosocial stress

Examination
- ask patient to show site of pain
- spasm of paraspinal muscles
- spinal tenderness/scoliosis/abnormal shape
- if leg symptoms, check straight-leg raising – record angles

Tests
- not necessary. Patients who expect an X-ray should be gently told that it will be of no help in finding the cause of their pain, and that the dose of radiation required is 120 times that of a chest X-ray. Scans are only indicated if a particular condition is suspected, e.g. vertebral fracture or metastasis

Self-care
- reassure the patient that most back pain is not serious and will get better without treatment
- the patient's emotional health plays a major part in the resolution of their back pain, and it is very important that health professionals convey a positive attitude from the beginning
- correct any misunderstandings about the meaning of the pain
- address mental health problems. Explain that stress causes muscular tension
- reducing activity may delay recovery
- encourage gentle mobilisation (activity within the limits of pain as soon as possible)
- if mattress over 10 years old, consider buying a new one

- discuss analgesics. If the patient pays prescription charges, ibuprofen and paracetamol are cheaper if bought OTC and can be used together up to the maximum daily dose. Combination analgesics containing codeine are also available OTC, but to obtain additional analgesia from codeine it is necessary to take at least 25 mg per dose, and many common combinations contain suboptimal doses. Suggest that the patient discusses this with the pharmacist:
  - ibuprofen (or naproxen prescribed, if ibuprofen ineffective)
  - paracetamol
  - codeine prescribed separately as codeine phosphate 30 mg tablets, if necessary (NB: this may cause constipation, which may be difficult to manage when patient has back pain – consider preventative medication)
- Download back care booklet from the Arthritis Research UK website (www. arthritisresearchuk.org) but explain that back pain is not caused by arthritis!
- consider buying a TENS machine
- recommend manipulation if pain not improving after 3 weeks and available/affordable

 Refer to doctor
- urgently if:
  - numbness/tingling in perianal area, bladder or bowel dysfunction (cauda equina syndrome, extremely rare)
  - sudden onset of severe pain with:
    - abdominal pain, discolouration of legs or stiffness (possible dissection of aortic aneurysm)
    - back stiffness (subarachnoid haemorrhage)
  - osteoporosis or cancer risk
  - sudden onset of severe pain over a vertebra, tender on examination and relieved by lying down (spinal fracture/metastasis)
  - pain remains when lying down, or disturbs sleep
  - thoracic pain
  - analgesics ineffective/severe muscle spasm (diazepam may be helpful)
- routinely if:
  - severe symptoms
  - sciatica (pain/numbness/tingling in one leg extending below the knee) not resolving after 3 weeks
  - aged < 20 years or > 50 years

References

Arthritis Research UK. *Back Pain*. Chesterfield: Arthritis Research UK; 2011. Available at: www. arthritisresearchuk.org/pdf/2002-Back-pain.pdf (accessed 8 December 2011).

Kendrick D, Fielding K, Bentley E, *et al*. Radiography of the lumbar spine in primary care patients with low back pain: randomized controlled trial. *BMJ*. 2001; 322: 400–5.

National Collaborating Centre for Primary Care. (2009) *Low Back Pain: early management of persistent non-specific low back pain. NICE guideline 88*. London: NIHCE; 2009. www.nice. org.uk/guidance/CG88

Welsh Medicines Reource Centre (WeMeReC). Management of acute low back pain. *WeMeReC Bulletin*. February 2008. Avaialable at: www.wemerec.org

Managing pain

Non-steroidal anti-inflammatory drugs

- contraindications to NSAIDs:
  - history of peptic ulcer or GI bleed
  - renal failure (eGFR < 30 mL/min)
  - severe liver failure
  - severe heart failure
  - taking prophylactic aspirin or warfarin
  - inflammatory bowel disease
  - pregnancy or trying to conceive
  - history of hypersensitivity to aspirin or any other NSAID
  - acute herpes virus infections (chickenpox, shingles, cold sores)
- use NSAIDs with caution if:
  - older and male. GI risk doubles with every decade above 55 years:
    - 1 per 1000 people per year at 55
    - 2 per 1000 people at 65
    - 4 per 1000 people at 75
  - hypertension
  - ischaemic heart disease
  - systemic lupus erythematosus
  - breastfeeding
  - asthma
  - recovering from surgery, fracture or injury
- NICE recommends co-prescribing a proton pump inhibitor (PPI), e.g. omeprazole 20 mg daily, to all patients over 45 given an NSAID for more than a short course, and it should be considered even for short courses if the patient is at high GI risk

References

National Collaborating Centre for Primary Care. *Low Back Pain: early management of persistent non-specific low back pain. NICE guideline 88*. London: NIHCE; 2009. www.nice.org.uk/guidance/CG88

Prodigy. *Clinical topic: Nonsteroidal anti-inflammatory drugs (standard or coxibs) – prescribing issues*. 2011. Available at: http://prodigy.clarity.co.uk/nsaids_prescribing_issues (accessed 29 January 2011).

6

Skin

Nurses often find skin problems daunting at first. Remember two important principles, which apply equally to all types of minor illness:

- find out and address the patient's agenda. This is commonly:
  — is it meningitis?
  — is it contagious?
  — (for an isolated lesion) is it cancer?
- take a good history. *This is where to find the diagnosis – your examination is for confirmation.* The four most useful questions are:
  — duration
  — fever/malaise
  — distribution – and is it symmetrical?
  — itch

Caution
- in darkly pigmented skin, it is difficult to assess the degree of inflammation

It may be helpful to compare the patient's rash with pictures. Dermnet (www.dermnetnz.org) or Dermis (www.dermis.net) are good online resources, or use one of the many books available.

It is quite likely that you will not be able to make a definite diagnosis. Provided that you have addressed the patient's concerns and ruled out serious illness, this does not matter. If the problem does not resolve, then the patient should be asked to make an appointment with a doctor.

Reference
Ashton R, Leppard B. *Differential Diagnosis in Dermatology*. Oxford: Radcliffe; 2004.

Rashes

History
- duration
- unwell: fever/malaise
- distribution

- itching
- did all spots appear at same time, or sequentially
- is rash constant, spreading, or coming and going
- previous episodes
- any contacts who are itching
- any new medication

Examination
- distribution/symmetry
- discrete (separate) or confluent (merging)
- colour
- surface – feel with fingertips
- are the areas:
  — weal-like (irregular, raised, blotchy)
  — flat (macules) or raised (papules)
  — containing fluid (vesicles)
- for itchy rashes, are burrows visible on the hands?

Now see the different sections:
A Acute generalized itchy rash
B Rash in a seriously ill patient
C Rash in a febrile patient
D Purple rashes
E Localised rashes
F Localised bacterial infections
G Miscellaneous

A. Acute generalized itchy rash:

1 chickenpox
2 urticaria
3 scabies
4 pityriasis rosea
5 eczema (*see* page 83)

1. Chickenpox
- caused by the herpes zoster virus
- incubation period 10–21 days
- significant exposure is 5 min face-to-face or 15 min in same room
- fever, headache and malaise, more marked in adults
- separate itchy papules at different stages of development, turning to blisters

Self-care

- calamine or crotamiton lotion OTC (keep in fridge) are often used to reduce itching
- chlorphenamine is useful at night because of its sedative action, but sedation may be unacceptable
- non-sedating antihistamines are probably ineffective
- avoid ibuprofen (see below)

Action

- prescribe high-dose aciclovir to the immunosuppressed, and consider it for ill adults and adolescents (14+ yr) who present within 24 h, especially if smoker or lactating
- for contacts who are pregnant, immunosuppressed or a baby under 4 weeks, check antibody status and contact microbiologist to consider zoster immunoglobulin (ZIG)
- notify Health Protection Unit in Scotland and Northern Ireland

Refer to doctor

- urgently if:
  - — immunosuppressed
  - — breathless/confused/severe headache/petechial rash
  - — pregnant/less than 4 weeks after childbirth
  - — baby aged under 4 weeks (30% mortality)

Cautions

- chickenpox may rarely be complicated by pneumonia, thrombocytopenia or encephalitis; pregnant women are at highest risk
- secondary bacterial infection is often suspected when chickenpox lesions become inflamed, but is surprisingly rare. The risk is increased if the patient is treated with an NSAID such as ibuprofen. If the lesions become painful, rather than itchy, if they weep any purulent fluid, or if a second phase of fever develops, then a secondary infection may indeed be present. Take a swab from any weeping lesion for bacterial culture, and give both flucloxacillin and amoxicillin to cover not only staphylococcus (the common skin pathogen) but also streptococcus, which has been implicated in life-threatening secondary infections following chickenpox.

Reference

[No authors listed]. Varicella, herpes zoster and nonsteroidal anti-inflammatory drugs: serious cutaneous complications [review]. *Prescribe Int.* **19**(106): 72–3.

Prodigy. *Clinical topic: Chickenpox.* 2011. Available at: http://prodigy.clarity.co.uk/chickenpox (accessed 29 August 2011).

Swingler G. Chickenpox. London: *BMJ*; 2007. Available at: www.clinicalevidence.com

2. Urticaria

This is a rash triggered by the immune system either appropriately (infection) or inappropriately (allergy), or for an unknown reason (idiopathic). It is caused by dilation of capillaries and the release of histamine from mast cells, causing leakage of plasma into the skin.

- common causes include:
  — drugs (e.g. aspirin, antibiotics)
  — viral infection
  — food allergy (especially lactose in babies)
  — bites and stings
  — heat or cold
  — vigorous exercise
  — pressure
  — alcohol
  — psychosocial stress
- also called 'nettle rash' (the botanical name of nettles is *Urtica*)
- itchy
- raised pale weals on a red/pink background (flare)
- check for tongue and lip swelling/wheeze/hypotension

Self-care
- oral (not topical) antihistamines: cetirizine or loratadine

Action
- if above ineffective, change to fexofenadine
- chlorphenamine may be added if sedation desirable/acceptable
- ranitidine may also be added (unlicensed indication)

Refer to doctor
- urgently if:
  — any suspicion of angio-oedema or anaphylaxis
  — antihistamines ineffective (to consider oral prednisolone, 40 mg/day for adults, or ranitidine)
- routinely if:
  — drug allergy suspected
  — symptoms recurrent

Reference
Grattan C, Powell S, Humphreys F, *et al*. Management and diagnostic guidelines for urticaria and angio-oedema. *Brit J Dermatol*. 2001; **144**(4): 708–14.

3. Scabies
- caused by a mite which burrows under the skin, most commonly on the hands
- widespread severe itching, worse at night. May affect the nipples or scrotum
- rash rarely on face in adults
- sleeping partners or other family members may be affected
- not acquired from domestic pets
- burrows may be visible on hands, or elsewhere – bumpy grey lines about 2–15 mm long
- spreading variable allergic rash develops after 4–6 weeks

Self-care

- permethrin dermal cream should be applied to all household and sexual contacts, repeated after 7 days
- a prescription is required for babies aged under 6 months
- apply to the whole body from the chin and ears downwards
- immunosuppressed, elderly or babies: treatment should also be applied to the face and scalp, avoiding the eye area
- be sure to cover finger and toe webs, and under nails
- do not apply just after a bath or shower
- wash off after 12 h
- reapply treatment if washed off before this time (e.g. to hands)
- machine wash clothes, towels, and bedding (at 50°C or above) on day of treatment
- sedative antihistamines (e.g. chlorphenamine) give best relief of itch, but sedation may be unacceptable
- it is debatable whether non-sedating antihistamines are effective
- *itching may persist for 6 weeks* after mites have been eradicated
- crotamiton may help

Caution

- children under two should be treated under medical supervision

Reference

Johnston G, Sladden M. Scabies: diagnosis and treatment. *BMJ*. 2005; **331**(7517): 619–22.

4. Pityriasis rosea

- occurs mainly in adolescents and young adults, and more often during autumn or spring
- malaise, fever or lymphadenopathy before the rash appeared
- usually a larger initial 'herald' patch, often on trunk, up to 2 weeks before
- numerous, widespread, salmon-coloured, oval patches, 1–2 cm
- ring of scaling just inside the edge
- appears over a period of days
- patches line up along the dermatome lines (*see* Figure 6.1), trunk and proximal limbs ('Christmas tree' rash in the T-shirt and shorts area)
- itching often present, usually mild but occasionally intense
- cause is not known, though herpes virus 6 and 7 have been implicated

Self-care

- new crops may occur for several weeks
- rash will last 6–12 weeks then disappear, leaving no trace
- in dark-skinned people, the marks may take longer to fade
- not contagious
- unlikely to recur
- emollients for itching (e.g. hydrous ointment)
- hydrocortisone ointment if itching severe

Reference

Prodigy. *Clinical topic: Pityriasis rosea*. 2011. Available at: http://prodigy.clarity.co.uk/pityriasis_rosea (accessed 29 August 2011).

B. Rash in a seriously ill patient

1 measles
2 meningococcal septicaemia
3 exotic disease (remember the travel history)

1. Measles

- uncommon, but increasing thanks to the MMR scare (374 confirmed cases in the UK in 2010). Any contacts?
- unlikely if two MMR vaccinations given
- 1–4 days of malaise, loss of appetite, nasal discharge before rash develops
- high fever and malaise
- cough
- conjunctivitis
- photophobia

Examination

- Koplik's spots may appear just before the rash; blue-grey specks like grains of salt with a red base on the buccal mucosa (inner cheeks)
- bright red maculopapular (flat and raised) areas which coalesce then peel
- rash starts on face and moves down the body
- check ears for otitis media

Self-care

- infectious for 4 days
- recovery may take 10 days
- take ibuprofen or paracetamol if needed for muscular pains
- drink adequate fluids
- wash hands frequently, avoid sharing cutlery, cups and towels; put used tissues in bin immediately

Action

- notify Health Protection Unit (HPU)
- refer to doctor if severe illness
- antibiotics may be needed for secondary otitis media or chest infection
- saliva tests will probably be requested later to confirm the diagnosis

References

Prodigy. *Clinical topic: Measles*. 2011. Available at: http://prodigy.clarity.co.uk/measles (accessed 29 August 2011).

World Health Organization. *Immunisation Monitoring*. 2011. Available at: http://apps.who. int/immunization_monitoring/en/globalsummary/timeseries/tsincidencemea.htm (accessed 5 February 2011).

2. *Meningococcal septicaemia*

- rare but important *as most will first present in primary care*
- high mortality
- patient looks ill, often drowsy or confused
- fever
- diarrhoea is a common early feature
- the classic rash is purpuric (i.e. dull purplish-red macules that do not blanch on pressure using a glass) but there may be a non-specific rash in the early stages
- low blood pressure, prolonged CRT, rapid pulse

Refer to doctor

- immediately for intravenous benzylpenicillin and transfer to hospital by emergency ambulance. If venous access difficult, give intramuscularly first and then attempt IV

C. Rash in a febrile patient

1 non-specific viral infection
2 slapped cheek (parvovirus B19)
3 hand, foot and mouth disease
4 scarlet fever

1. *Nonspecific viral infection*

Many viruses cause a diffuse macular rash. There are thousands of different types of virus, and the type of rash that they cause is not consistent, so it is usually impossible to name the virus. It may reassure the patient or parent to know if there have been similar cases in the neighbourhood. Some specific syndromes such as roseola infantum have been described, but in the absence of any specific treatment, such labels are not usually helpful. It does not usually matter that you cannot identify the virus, unless the patient is pregnant or has been in contact with a pregnant woman. Rubella is now rare; there were only 9 confirmed cases in the UK in 2010. Parvovirus is much more common.

Examination

- check for pharyngitis (possible scarlet fever, *see* page 71)

Self-care

- no specific treatment available
- no exclusion from school needed

Refer to doctor

- urgently if pregnant

References

Health Protection Agency. *Guidance on Viral Rash in Pregnancy*. London: Health Protection Agency; 2011. www.hpa.org.uk/Topics/InfectiousDiseases/InfectionsAZ/Pregnancy (accessed 30 November 2011).

World Health Organization. *Immunisation Monitoring*. 2011. Available at: http://apps.who.int/immunization_monitoring/en/globalsummary/timeseries/tsincidencerub.htm (accessed 5 February 2011).

2. Slapped cheek

- known as erythema infectiosum or fifth disease
- commonest in children aged 4–10
- caused by parvovirus B19
- bright red cheeks
- maybe fever, nasal discharge, diarrhoea
- later maybe lacy rash on trunk and limbs
- joint pains in adults
- immunosuppressed patient may develop bone marrow problems

Self-care

- no specific treatment available
- no exclusion from school needed
- take paracetamol or ibuprofen for joint pain

Refer to doctor

- urgently if:
  — pregnant (may cause miscarriage)
  — immunosuppressed
  — blood disorders

The last two groups of patients will need FBC and reticulocyte count, also serology (in consultation with microbiologist).

References

Prodigy. *Clinical topic: Parvovirus B19 infection*. 2011. Available at: http://prodigy.clarity.co.uk/parvovirus_b19_infection (accessed 29 August 2011).

Health Protection Agency. *Guidance on Viral Rash in Pregnancy*. London: Health Protection Agency; 2011. www.hpa.org.uk/Topics/InfectiousDiseases/InfectionsAZ/Pregnancy/ (accessed 30 November 2011).

3. Hand, foot and mouth disease

- caused by a virus (usually coxsackie A16)
- mainly affects children under 10
- fever, sore throat and malaise

- painful blisters in mouth, then hands and feet
- not related to foot and mouth disease in animals

Self-care
- no specific treatment available
- no exclusion from school needed
- take paracetamol for pain
- watch fluid intake and seek help if dehydration suspected

Reference
Prodigy. *Clinical topic: Hand, foot and mouth disease.* 2011. http://prodigy.clarity.co.uk/hand_foot_and_mouth_disease (accessed 28 November 2011).

4. Scarlet fever
- caused by group A streptococcus
- 4000 notifications in 2008/9
- commonest in children (peak age 4)
- sore throat/cervical lymphadenopathy
- fever and malaise
- nausea and vomiting
- blanching rough red pinpricks, starting on abdomen and chest, peeling after 7 days
- flushed face, pale around the mouth
- skin folds deep red in colour
- red throat with macules over the hard and soft palate
- complications are rare; secondary infections (e.g. pneumonia), late complications (e.g. rheumatic fever, glomerulonephritis)

Self-care
- scarlet fever is not usually serious nowadays
- infectious for 24 h after starting antibiotics: especially avoid contact with immunosuppressed people or those with heart valve problems
- wash hands frequently, avoid sharing cutlery, cups and towels; put used tissues in bin immediately

Action
- prescribe amoxicillin in children or phenoxymethylpenicillin in adults
- notify HPU

Refer to doctor
- urgently if
  — heart valve disease
  — immunosuppressed

D. Purple rashes

Purple rashes are usually caused by extravasation of blood from the vessels just under the skin, therefore they do not blanch on pressure or when covered by a glass (the 'tumbler test'). Pinpoint rashes are described as petechial, larger areas as purpuric. Such rashes may be caused by:

- pressure changes, e.g. attempted strangulation, violent vomiting, 'love bites'
- meningococcal septicaemia
- blood or clotting abnormalities, e.g. leukaemia, thrombocytopenia, aspirin in the elderly
- vasculitis, e.g. Henoch-Schönlein purpura, which mainly affects children

Refer to doctor

- *urgently*, unless obviously due to pressure changes

E. Localised rashes

1   cold sores
2   shingles
3   warts and verrucae
4   molluscum contagiosum
5   fungal infections
6   nappy rash

1. Cold sores

Caused by recurrence of herpes simplex virus (HSV-1).

History

- often recurrent on same site (not always the lip)
- tingling in skin before appearance of the sore
- triggers include stress, UV light, premenstruation, minor trauma to the area of the cold sore and other infections like colds

Examination

- blisters on the border of the lip, tongue or mouth which break down into small red areas with yellowish membrane
- check for evidence of cellulitis (*see* page 81)

Self-care

- aciclovir cream if within 48 h of appearance (not in pregnancy)
- do not share objects which have touched the area
- take care not to touch eyes or genitalia after touching cold sore
- sunblock may help prevention
- avoid contact with babies under 4 weeks old until sore has healed (risk of herpes simplex encephalitis)

Refer to doctor

- urgently if:
  — baby under 4 weeks
  — immunosuppressed
  — severe (may need oral aciclovir)
- routinely if:
  — recurrent cold sores

Reference

Prodigy. *Clinical topic: Herpes simplex – oral*. 2011. Available at: http://prodigy.clarity.co.uk/ herpes_simplex_oral (accessed 29 August 2011).

2. Shingles

Caused by recurrence of herpes zoster virus, maybe after a period of debility or psychosocial stress. More common and more likely to cause long-term pain in those over 60.

History

- affects area of skin supplied by one nerve root (*see* Figure 6.1)
- therefore, only one side of the body is affected
- malaise, mild fever and burning or tingling pain may occur up to 4 days before
- is patient immunosuppressed or pregnant?

Examination

- affects the area of skin supplied by one nerve root (dermatome) (commonest on the chest)
- starts with macules and papules which develop into painful blisters weeping infectious fluid
- they crust over after 2–4 weeks
- note which nerve root is affected (*see* Figure 6.1)
- if face affected, check whether rash involves the tip of nose or eye
- local lymph nodes may be enlarged

Self-care

- keep the rash dry
- creams and lotions are best avoided because of the risk of spreading skin bacteria into the blistered area
- avoid contact with newborn infants, pregnant women who have not had chickenpox and immunosuppressed
- fluid from the rash may infect someone else with chickenpox, but not with shingles. However, the risk of infection is very low if the rash is covered, and routine exclusion from school and work is not necessary
- malaise may require rest and time off work
- seek advice again if the rash 'flares up' or fever develops (because of secondary infection)
- paracetamol (not ibuprofen) for initial pain

Prescription

- aciclovir tablets 800 mg, five times daily for 10 days if:
  — immunosuppressed
  — nose or eye affected
- aciclovir tablets 800 mg, five times daily for 7 days if within 72 h of onset if:
  — aged over 50
  — affecting area other than the trunk
  — severe symptoms

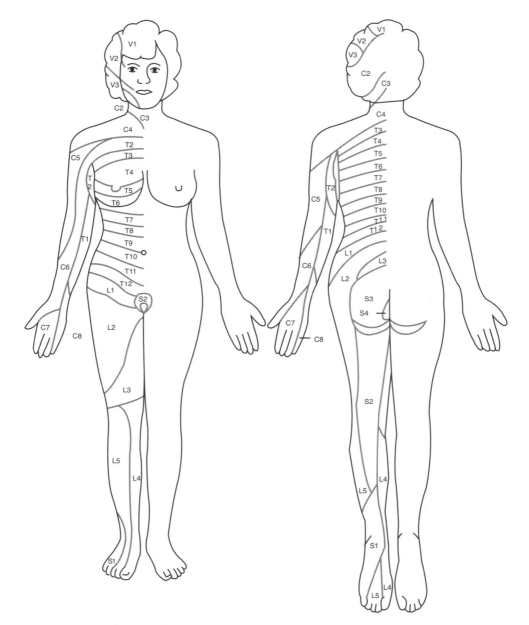

FIGURE 6.1 Dermatome diagram. Each area is labelled with the spinal nerve that carries sensation from the skin to the spinal cord. The areas overlap to some extent, and an individual person may vary from normal.

C, cervical; L, lumbar; S, sacral; T, thoracic; V, fifth cranial nerve (trigeminal)

Refer to doctor
- urgently if:
  — nose or eye affected (for eye clinic referral)
  — immunosuppressed patient with severe symptoms
  — pregnant
  — pain troublesome despite simple analgesia (may need medicines for neuropathic pain)

Reference

Dworkin RH, Johnson RW, Breuer J, *et al*. Recommendations for the management of herpes zoster. *Clin Infect Dis*. 2007; **44**(Suppl. 1): S1–26.

3. Warts and verrucae
- raised pale swellings, maybe with a surface like a cauliflower
- flattened areas with underlying black dots (verrucae)
- caused by a virus

Self-care
- contagious – take steps to avoid self- or cross-infection. A patient with a verruca should use a waterproof plaster for swimming and sports, and avoid sharing a towel
- most disappear by themselves with time, but may take 2–3 years
- remove hard skin with an emery board
- no treatment is the best option
- salicylic acid (OTC):
  — appears to be the most effective treatment, from the limited evidence available. Proper application is important:
    – soak in warm water for 5–10 minutes
    – avoid applying the treatment to the surrounding skin
    – do not apply to the face
    – do not use in people with diabetes
- liquid nitrogen:
  — not for children under the age of 10
  — not suitable for people with diabetes, poor circulation or reduced sensation
  — may also cause dramatic blood blistering, temporary numbness and scarring
- duct tape:
  — cover the wart with duct tape for 6 days
  — if tape falls off, apply a fresh piece
  — remove tape, soak wart in water, and debride with emery board
  — leave the wart uncovered overnight and apply a fresh piece of tape next day
  — continue treatment for up to 2 months
- banana skin:
  — anecdotally, the application of a banana skin, with the white inside part taped against the wart, each night for 2 weeks has often been reported to be effective – but it seems highly unlikely that a clinical trial on this treatment would ever be funded. It does have the advantage of being virtually free, with no known side-effects

Refer to doctor
- routinely:
  — anogenital warts
  — single wart in the elderly (may be a squamous carcinoma)

Reference
Gibbs S, Harvey I. Topical treatments for cutaneous warts. *Cochrane Database Syst Rev.* 2006; **3**: CD001781.

4. Molluscum contagiosum
This is a poxvirus infection which produces clusters of round, raised, pearly white lesions (sometimes with a darker central dimple) usually on the trunk and limbs of children. It is best left untreated as it resolves completely, without scarring, after several months. If itching is a problem, treat with emollients or hydrocortisone ointment. Sometimes secondary bacterial infection may occur.

Reference
Van der Wouden JC, Menke J, Gajadin S, *et al*. Interventions for cutaneous molluscum contagiosum. *Cochrane Database Syst Rev.* 2006; **2**: CD004767.

5. Fungal infections (tinea)
- of the foot (athlete's foot)
- of the flexures
- of the body ('ringworm')
- of the nails

History
- itchy red rash, slowly spreading
- not usually symmetrical
- treatments previously tried

Examination
- eczema-like patches
- often a scaly, inflamed edge
- central area may appear normal
- in toe webs, under breasts (intertrigo), in groin

Self-care
- explain that it is an infection acquired from other humans or animals
- wash the affected area daily and dry thoroughly
- wash clothes, towels and bed linen frequently
- wear loose-fitting clothes made of cotton or a material designed to wick moisture away from the skin

- miconazole cream applied twice daily for 3 weeks
- if clotrimazole or miconazole tried and ineffective, use terbinafine cream for 1 week. If both have failed, try undecenoic acid (Mycota, OTC)

Refer to doctor

- routinely if rash persists despite an adequate course of treatment (may need oral terbinafine)

Reference

Health Protection Agency. *Fungal Skin and Nail Infections: diagnosis and laboratory investigation. Quick reference guide for primary care*. London: Health Protection Agency; 2009. Available at: www.hpa.org.uk/Topics/InfectiousDiseases/InfectionsAZ/PrimaryCareGuidance/ (accessed 16 December 2011).

6. Nappy rash

History

- duration
- creams tried
- other areas affected (makes nappy rash unlikely)

Examination

- red and shiny or scaly areas, not involving the groin
- check for satellite spots
- look for oral thrush

Self-care

- leave nappy off when possible
- clean and change nappy as soon as wet or soiled
- use water, or fragrance-free and alcohol-free baby wipes
- dry gently after cleaning — avoid vigorous rubbing
- bathe once daily
- do not use soap or bath additives
- use high-absorbency nappies
- barrier creams such as Metanium, applied at each nappy change

Prescription

- fungal superinfection is common in nappy rash which has been present for more than 48 h. The presence of satellite spots and the involvement of the skin creases make this more likely. If suspected, recommend clotrimazole cream for 2–3 weeks and avoiding barrier cream
- if severe, also use hydrocortisone ointment for the first week

Refer to doctor or health visitor

- if not responding to treatment

Reference

Prodigy. *Clinical topic: Nappy rash*. 2011. Available at: http://prodigy.clarity.co.uk/nappy_rash (accessed 29 August 2011).

F. Localised bacterial infections

1 impetigo
2 boils
3 cellulitis
4 ingrowing toenail
5 bites
6 stings

1. Impetigo

- golden crusted lesions, usually caused by staphylococcus, sometimes streptococcus
- commonly on faces of children, though may occur elsewhere
- may be secondary to wound or viral lesion
- patient may be systemically unwell if infection is severe
- bullous impetigo (blistering and painful) is uncommon; neonates are most often affected

Self-care

- wash off crusts with soapy water
- stay off school until lesions crusted, or for 48 h after starting treatment
- use own facecloth and towel
- seek help if worsening, or no improvement after 4 days

Prescription

- topical sodium fusidate ointment if localised
- consider treating inside nostrils, if recurrent facial impetigo
- mupirocin should be reserved for the treatment of MRSA
- oral flucloxacillin if extensive or severe (clarithromycin if the patient is allergic to
- penicillin)

Reference

Koning S, Verhagen AP, Van Suijlekom-Smit LWA, *et al*. Interventions for impetigo. *Cochrane Database Syst Rev*. 2004; **2**: CD003261.

2. Boils

History

- duration
- fever
- symptoms of diabetes: thirst/polyuria/tiredness
- immunosuppressed

Examination

- fluctuation (sensation of fluid moving between two fingers placed on either side – imagine a balloon full of water)
- cellulitis
- enlarged lymph nodes (suggest underlying cellulitis)

Tests

- if recurrent boils, consider:
  — nasal swab for staphylococci
  — FBC
  — FBG
  — HIV serology

Self-care

- apply heat to encourage pointing (e.g. warm flannel) four times daily
- cover with sterile dressing

Action

- magnesium sulphate paste is traditionally used, although there is no evidence to support it
- incise and drain if fluctuant

Antibiotics for boils

Prescribe an antibiotic if:
- unwell with fever or cellulitis
- high-risk group (immunosuppressed, diabetes)
- on the face

Antibiotic choice

- flucloxacillin for 7 days
- clarithromycin if the patient is allergic to penicillin

Refer to doctor

- urgently if:
  — facial boil causing cellulitis (can be life-threatening)
  — apparent boil in anogenital area or natal cleft (between buttocks) – may be Bartholin's cyst, Crohn's disease or pilonidal abscess

Reference

Prodigy. *Clinical topic: Boils, carbuncles, and staphylococcal carriage.* 2011. Available at: http://prodigy.clarity.co.uk/boils_carbuncles_and_staphylococcal_carriage/management (accessed 29 August 2011).

Screening for diabetes

Much has been written about this, and there will be a protocol for your area based on the international criteria for the diagnosis and the characteristics of the various tests for diabetes. The protocol might start with a fasting blood glucose level as the first step, but screening whole populations in this way is burdensome and not as effective as targeting those at higher risk of diabetes. But how do you decide who is at high risk?

- High risk: if you strongly suspect diabetes because of classic symptoms, such as thirst, polyuria and weight loss, then formal testing with fasting blood glucose/HbA1c/glucose tolerance test is needed. Follow your protocol
- Moderate risk: if the patient is at high risk of having diabetes but has no symptoms, it is also appropriate to follow the usual protocol. For a list of risk factors, see www.diabetes. org.uk/Guide-to-diabetes/Introduction-to-diabetes/ Causes_and_Risk_Factors
- Low risk: if the patient has a minor illness known to be more common in those with diabetes, such as cystitis or boils, but has no symptoms of diabetes, then test the urine for glucose. If this proves positive, then it is quite likely that the patient does indeed have diabetes, but this needs confirming with blood tests. If the urine is negative for glucose, this does not completely exclude diabetes (the elderly in particular may not show glucose in the urine despite fairly high blood levels), but the test is adequate when the chance of finding diabetes is low.

Testing the urine for glucose is useful in primary care when the individual's risk of diabetes is low. The test is quick, inexpensive, does not require the patient to fast and the result is known immediately. Positive results need further investigation to establish the diagnosis.

Reference

World Health Organization. *Screening for Type 2 Diabetes*. 2003. Available at: www.who.int/diabetes/publications/en/screening_mnc03. pdf (accessed 29 August 2011).

3. Cellulitis

A bacterial infection of the deeper layers of the skin, usually caused by *Streptococcus pyogenes* (two thirds of cases) or *Staphylococcus aureus* (one third of cases).

History
- duration
- nature of wound
- fever/malaise
- pain
- tetanus status
- immunosuppressed (especially intravenous substance use and diabetes)

Examination
- temperature
- discharge
- cellulitis: red, hot, swollen, hard, tender area, with possible blisters
- tracking (lymphangitis)
- lymphadenopathy

Tests
- take swab if discharge from a significant wound
- if history of recurrent skin infections, or symptoms or family history of diabetes, consider FBG

Self-care
- keep limb elevated (if applicable)
- mark boundary with indelible pen
- seek help if area is enlarging
- take paracetamol for pain
- use an emollient, e.g. hydrous ointment, after 48 h

Action
- wound cleaning and dressing as appropriate
- consider Revaxis booster
- antibiotics for 7–10 days (longer in lymphoedema)
- review after 7 days (sooner if concerned)

TABLE 6.1 Antibiotic choice for cellulitis

Presentation	Antibiotic	Penicillin allergy
Typical cellulitis	Flucloxacillin (high dose)	Clarithromycin
Seawater injury	Flucloxacillin + doxycycline	Clarithromycin + doxycycline
Freshwater injury	Flucloxacillin + ciprofloxacin	Clarithromycin + ciprofloxacin
Facial cellulitis	Co-amoxiclav	Seek advice

Refer to doctor
- urgently for consideration of hospital admission if:
  — child under 1 year
  — severe infection
  — lymphangitis
  — worsening despite treatment
  — immunosuppressed
  — high-risk patients (heart valve problem, pacemaker, artificial joint)
  — diabetes
  — pointing abscess (for incision and drainage)
  — on face (may need admission)
  — in anogenital area or natal cleft (between buttocks)
  — not responding to initial treatment after 3 days
  — tracking

Reference
Clinical Resource Efficiency Support Team (CREST). *Guidelines on the Management of Cellulitis in Adults*. Belfast: Clinical Resource Efficiency Support Team; 2005. Available at: www.gain-ni. org/Library/Guidelines/cellulitis-guide.pdf (accessed 8 February 2011).

4. Ingrowing toenail
History
- duration
- discharge
- previous episodes
- diabetes

Examination
- cellulitis
- inflammation where the nail digs in is expected, but pus, spreading redness or fever indicate cellulitis
- discharge
- granulation tissue

Test
- swab if discharge

Self-care
- soak toe in warm salty water for 10 minutes (1 teaspoon of salt in 500 mL water)
- with cotton bud, push skin fold over ingrown nail, down and away from the nail. Start at root of the nail and move outwards
- repeat daily for a few weeks
- as end of nail grows forward, push tiny pledget of cotton wool under it to help nail grow over skin

- change cotton wool daily
- allow nail to grow forward until clear of end of toe
- cut nail straight across
- see chiropodist if persistent/recurrent
- keep feet clean and dry
- let air get to toes when possible
- avoid tight shoes
- use cotton socks rather than synthetic

Action
- if localised cellulitis (pus, fever, spreading redness):
  — flucloxacillin for 7 days (or clarithromycin if allergic to penicillin)

Refer to doctor
- urgently if:
  — immunosuppressed with cellulitis
  — diabetes with cellulitis

Reference
Dermnet NZ. *Ingrown Toenails*. 2009. Available at: www.dermnetnz.org/hair-nails-sweat/onychocryptosis.html (accessed 8 February 2011).

G. Miscellaneous
1 eczema
2 seborrhoeic dermatitis
3 head lice
4 suspected skin cancer
5 acne

1. Eczema
This condition accounts for 30% of all skin consultations in primary care. It occurs when the lipid layer which covers the skin becomes thin, causing water loss. Emotional or environmental factors may trigger a flare. The term 'dermatitis' is used for eczema due to a known allergen.

History
- duration
- previous episodes
- suspected cause (e.g. solvents, nickel, detergents, latex)
- distribution (usually symmetrical, in flexures, face, hands)
- itching
- fever/discharge/pain (suggest infection)
- previous treatments and effects
- occupation (hairdressers are at high risk)

Examination
- poorly defined pink scaly patches
- maybe dry and cracking
- symmetrical
- scratch marks/damage
- is it infected/inflamed/weeping

Tests
- swab if discharging
- scrapings for fungus if diagnosis in doubt, or treatment unsuccessful

Self-care
- treatments will control but not cure
- avoid scratching – rub with fingertips or soft paintbrush
- keep cool
- if hands affected, use cotton-lined rubber gloves for washing up
- dietary changes and dust mite avoidance are not recommended
- use emollients (sometimes called moisturisers) three or four times daily; do not rub in
- about 500 g of emollient per week may be needed
- consider trial sizes first, to avoid expensive mistakes
- ointments work better than creams, if stickiness tolerated
- hydrous ointment is the first choice: Cetraben or DiproBase are alternatives
- pump dispensers are preferred – if using pots, avoid contamination from fingers
- emollients may be flammable
- avoid detergents (e.g. bubble bath – even that marketed for babies)
- bath additives such as QV may be helpful, although their effectiveness is disputed. Shower preparations are not recommended
- use aqueous cream as a soap substitute
- if itching is troublesome, consider chlorphenamine, if sedation tolerated
- non-sedating antihistamines are unlikely to be effective
- if eczema is inflamed, use topical steroids (hydrocortisone or Eumovate) until redness has settled
- allow emollient to absorb before applying steroids

Action
- if not responding, reconsider diagnosis (may be fungal)
- if infected, give oral flucloxacillin, or clarithromycin if allergic to penicillin

Refer to doctor
- urgently if:
  - severe infection
  - widespread vesicles (eczema herpeticum)

Preparation	Steroid potency
Betnovate	High
Eumovate	Moderate
Hydrocortisone	Low
Emollients	Zero
Bath additives	Zero

FIGURE 6.2 Treatments for eczema.

Caution

- topical steroids stronger than hydrocortisone may cause atrophy and thinning of the skin after prolonged use. Tiny blood vessels become visible, for which no treatment is available. The skin of the face is the most sensitive, the palms and soles least sensitive. Children's skin is more sensitive than adults' – *do not use any stronger steroid than hydrocortisone in children, or on the face*
- 1% hydrocortisone cream can be bought OTC for considerably less than the prescription charge, but the packs carry warnings not to use the product in children or on the face, and the pharmacist is not allowed to sell them for these purposes. If the patient has been assessed by a clinician and a prescription isued, these warnings are unnecessary

References

[No authors listed]. Bath emollients for atopic eczema: why use them? *Drug Ther Bull.* 2007; **45**: 73–5.

Klein PA, Clark RA. An evidence-based review of the efficacy of antihistamines in relieving pruritus in atopic dermatitis. *Arch Dermatol.* 1999; **135**(12): 1522–5.

National Institute for Health and Clinical Excellence. *Atopic Eczema in Children: management of atopic eczema in children from birth up to the age of 12 years.* NICE guideline 57. London: NIHCE; 2007. www.nice.org.uk/guidance/CG57

Scottish Intercollegiate Guidelines Network (SIGN). *Management of Atopic Eczema in Primary Care: SIGN guideline 125.* Edinburgh: Scottish Intercollegiate Guidelines Network; 2011. www.sign.ac.uk/pdf/sign125.pdf

2. Seborrhoeic dermatitis

This is a type of skin inflammation which occurs in babies aged 2 weeks to 6 months, and also in adults. It is affected by hormone balance and stress, but the yeast *Malassezia* is also implicated.

- in adults: scalp (dandruff), nasolabial folds, ears, eyebrows and chest
- in infants: scalp (cradle cap), face, ears, neck and nappy area
- red, flaky, greasy patches which may be itchy

Self-care

- avoid alcohol-based cosmetics
- on the face, minimise use of soap and shaving cream

- use emollient soap substitutes, e.g aqueous cream, Hydromol Bath & Shower
- look for dietary triggers
- consider stress management
- on the scalp, apply warm olive oil or baby oil for several hours, then wash with Capasal shampoo and brush gently to remove scales. If problem persists, then use ketoconazole 2% shampoo
- on the face, use miconazole cream until the symptoms have settled

Action
- if self-care measures have failed, consider adding hydrocortisone 1% ointment or Canesten HC

Refer to doctor
- if simple measures are ineffective, to consider alternative antifungals and/or a stronger steroid application

References

O'Connor NR, McLaughlin MR, Ham P. Newborn skin: part I. Common rashes. *Am Fam Physician.* 2008; **77**(1): 47–52.

Schwartz RA, Janusz CA, Janniger CK. Seborrheic dermatitis: an overview. *Am Fam Physician.* 2006; **74**(1): 125–30.

3. Head lice
History
- nits
- lice
- scratching

Examination
- examine head for nits and live lice
- louse eggs adhere to hair tightly, whereas dandruff falls off easily
- look for enlarged occipital lymph nodes

Self-care
- check all of household and treat *only those in whom live lice have been found*
- wet combing with conditioner is the best method of checking, because it immobilizes the lice
- use one of the following methods:
  - dimethicone lotion – seems to have the best evidence of effectiveness
  - wet combing using the Bug Buster comb
  - coconut, anise and ylang-ylang spray (Lyclear SprayAway) (not for those with asthma)
  - malathion 0.5% aqueous liquid
- repeat according to method

- reassure – lice prefer clean hair
- warn patient that eggs will still be visible after treatment

Reference

Prodigy. *Clinical topic: Head lice*. 2011. Available at: http://prodigy.clarity.co.uk/head_lice (accessed 29 August 2011).

4. Suspected skin cancer

Most moles develop in early childhood and adolescence, and there is a gradual decrease in their number in old age. Not unreasonably, malignant melanoma is a concern behind many consultations, in which most patients need reassurance. Many so-called moles are in fact seborrhoeic keratoses which are superficial, golden brown in colour with a scaly, greasy surface. They are harmless. Not all skin cancers are pigmented: basal cell carcinomas (rodent ulcers) are pink or red lesions most commonly found on the face, whereas squamous cell carcinomas can arise anywhere on the body.

History
- patient's concerns
- duration
- enlarging/changing shape
- itch/change in sensation
- inflammation/oozing

Examination
- colour
- diameter
- feel for induration (hardness)
- edge – rolled?
- major features of mole (two points each):
  — change in size
  — irregular shape
  — irregular colour
- minor features of mole (one point each):
  — largest diameter 7 mm or more
  — inflammation
  — oozing
  — change in sensation

Self-care
- watch the area, maybe measure or photograph it, and seek help if you notice any of the following (ABCDE):
  — **A**symmetrical
  — **B**order irregular
  — **C**olours (more than one)

— Diameter (more than 6 mm)
— Evolving over time

Refer to doctor

- urgently if:
  — pigmented lesion with three or more points
  — any slow-growing lesion over 7 mm in diameter
- routinely if:
  — suspected basal cell carcinoma

Reference

National Collaborating Centre for Primary Care. *Referral Guidelines for Suspected Cancer: NICE guideline 27*. London: NIHCE; 2005. pp. 10–42. www.nice.org.uk/guidance/CG27

5. Acne vulgaris

History

- distribution
- previous treatments and results

Examination

- mild acne: blackheads (open comedones) and whiteheads (closed comedones)
- moderate acne: inflamed papules and pustules

Self-care

- there are many myths about acne – it is not infectious, or caused by poor hygiene. Diet does not affect it and sunlight does not improve it
- wash with soap and lukewarm water, just twice daily
- use lukewarm water
- do not scrub or pick at the skin
- avoid cosmetics as much as possible, and remove them completely at night
- if skin dry, use water-based emollient such as Cetraben
- benzoyl peroxide (PanOxyl) is the OTC treatment with the best evidence of effectiveness. Always start with 2.5% gel and only increase the strength if necessary, as there is evidence that this concentration is as effective as higher strengths

Prescription

- for mild acne with oily skin, tretinoin or benzoyl peroxide (PanOxyl, OTC) are first-line
- if these cause irritation, offer topical antibiotic (erythromycin as Zineryt) or azelaic acid
- if above treatment fails or acne inflamed, offer benzoyl peroxide with topical antibiotic (Duac)
- consider combined oral contraceptive (standard or co-cyprindiol). These should only be prescribed by a clinician with a family-planning qualification
- consider oxytetracycline if topical treatment fails, or if acne is moderate or severe
- for women, ensure adequate contraception if any oral tetracycline is prescribed

References

Arowojolu AO, Gallo MF, Lopez LM, *et al*. Combined oral contraceptive pills for treatment of acne. *Cochrane Database Syst Rev*. 2009; **3**: CD004425.

Bowman S, Gold M, Nasir A, *et al*. Comparison of clindamycin/benzoyl peroxide, tretinoin plus clindamycin, and the combination of clindamycin/benzoyl peroxide and tretinoin plus clindamycin in the treatment of acne vulgaris: a randomized, blinded study. *J Drugs Dermatol*. 2005; **4**(5): 611–18.

Magin P, Pond D, Smith W, *et al*. A systematic review of the evidence for 'myths and misconceptions' in acne management: diet, face-washing and sunlight. *Fam Pract*. 2005; **22**(1): 1–9.

7

Abdomen

Abdominal pain

History

- site
- duration
- intermittent/continuous
- stabbing/dull/colicky
- previous episodes (diagnosis and outcome)
- previous abdominal operations
- date of last menstrual period (LMP)/vaginal discharge or bleeding/contraception
- associated features:
  - fever
  - constipation/diarrhoea/blood or mucus in stool
  - vomiting/nausea/anorexia
  - dysuria/frequency
  - pain in testicles or groin
  - upper respiratory tract infection in children (may cause abdominal pain due to enlarged lymph nodes)
- OTC preparations tried

Examination

- examine abdomen, check groins for swelling
- record site of pain, any tenderness
- check for masses or distension
- examine tonsils in children

Tests

- test urine for protein/blood/glucose/nitrites
- send MSU for culture if low or unilateral pain, or urinary symptoms

Refer to doctor

- always, unless obvious gastro-enteritis or urinary tract infection (UTI) (see those protocols)
- urgently if:
  — severe
  — less than 1 week history
  — testicular pain or groin swelling

Caution

- ectopic pregnancy causes severe lower abdominal pain, usually one-sided, in a woman whose period is late or just due. She may collapse with the pain, particularly if a vaginal examination is attempted. If suspected, arrange pregnancy test and refer to doctor urgently

Dyspepsia

History

- what does the patient mean by the words they use?
- upper abdominal discomfort
- epigastric or right-sided location (suggests gallstones)
- feeling of fullness
- belching
- heartburn
- relation to meals and exercise
- smoking and alcohol
- diet (e.g. irregular meals, large meals at night, fatty foods, excessive citrus fruit juices can all cause digestive symptoms)
- psychosocial stress
- associated symptoms:
  — vomiting
  — bowel habit/motion colour
  — weight loss
- previous episodes, how treated
- OTC preparations tried
- medication, especially aspirin or other NSAID, warfarin, prednisolone, selective serotonin reuptake inhibitor (SSRI)

Examination

- examine abdomen
- record site of pain
- check for abnormal swellings

Tests
- arrange *Helicobacter pylori* test *before* prescribing any medication (should not be performed if patient has taken PPI, ranitidine or antibiotics in previous 2 weeks)
- consider FBC

Self-care
- if overweight, try to reduce
- if smoker, consider quitting
- if excessive alcohol intake, consider reducing
- stop any NSAID, unless taken for rheumatoid arthritis (in which case make appointment with doctor)
- *but* do not stop prophylactic aspirin – make appointment with doctor
- for mild symptoms, try antacids: Mucogel or Gaviscon Advance (both OTC)
- omeprazole and pantoprazole can be bought OTC but should not be used long term

Prescription
- omeprazole 20 mg daily for one month with appointment for review

Refer to doctor
- urgently if:
  — sudden onset or related to exercise (may be cardiac)
  — alarm symptoms:
    – difficulty in swallowing
    – gastrointestinal blood loss
    – persistent vomiting
    – unexplained significant weight loss
    – abdominal mass
- routinely if:
  — suspected gallstones
  — aged over 55
  — persistent/recurrent symptoms
  — patient is on medication listed under 'history'

Reference

Delaney BC, Qume M, Moayyedi P, *et al. Helicobacter pylori* test and treat versus proton pump inhibitor in initial management of dyspepsia in primary care: multicentre randomised controlled trial (MRC-CUBE trial). *BMJ.* 2008; **336**(7645): 651–4.

Diarrhoea and vomiting

History
- duration: preceding constipation
- severity: number of episodes in last 24 hours, stool consistency
- blood (red, brown or black) in motion/vomit

- fever
- fluid intake
- urine output
- contacts with similar symptoms, especially if they started on the same day
- hospital admission in previous 8 weeks
- broad-spectrum antibiotics in previous 8 weeks
- foreign travel
- suspect foods
- sorbitol (in diet foods, chewing gum) may cause diarrhoea
- possibility of pregnancy
- occupation – food handler/carer/health professional
- previous bowel disease
- immunosuppressed
- relevant medication which may have caused the symptoms, e.g. antibiotics, NSAIDs, metformin, laxatives
- relevant medication which will be affected by the illness, e.g. warfarin, anti-epileptic drugs, ACEIs, combined oral contraceptives (COC)
- PPIs such as omeprazole (increased risk of *Clostridium difficile* (*C. diff*))

Examination
- temperature
- dehydration
    - fontanelle in babies under 1 year
    - dry tongue/mouth
    - dry skin not reshaping after a soft pinch
    - sunken eyes
- pulse
- standing blood pressure in adults
- CRT in children
- abdominal examination
- consider rectal examination if overflow suspected (*see* 'Cautions')

Test
- stool culture if motions are still liquid and:
    - suspected food poisoning
    - febrile/systemically unwell
    - blood or pus in stool
    - immunosuppressed
    - recent broad-spectrum antibiotic therapy
    - recent hospital admission
    - recent travel to countries outside Europe/North America/Australia/New Zealand (also request ova, cysts and parasites if tropical area)
    - persistent watery diarrhoea after 7 days

- consider stool culture if:
  - food handler/carer/healthcare staff/in contact with vulnerable people (check with HPU)
  - pregnant
  - on PPI
  - recommended method: ask patient to collect 5 mL sample from clingfilm-lined container. Write patient's name on specimen bottle, or affix label, before giving out. Less than 5% of samples will identify a bacterial cause
- also check MSU in children under five with persistent or recurrent vomiting or diarrhoea (*see* page 104)

Self-care

- give reassurance: rarely serious in primary care
- dehydration is rare over 6 months of age (explain warning signs)
- take care when washing hands after using toilet/changing nappy
- remember to use the clean hand (i.e. not the one which has been used for wiping) to flush the toilet and turn on the taps
- toilet seats, handles, taps, and toilet door handles should be cleaned at least daily with hot water and detergent. Also use disinfectant or bleach to clean toilets
- soiled clothing should be washed separately at a minimum of 60°C
- do not return to work/school/day care until free of symptoms for 48 hours
- if *Cryptosporidium* diagnosed, do not swim in public pool for 2 weeks
- sip extra fluids, e.g. 200 mL for each loose stool in adults
- avoid fruit juices and fizzy drinks, but flat cold cola is a logical option (not the sugar-free type)
- supplement with oral rehydration solution (ORS) if:
  - child under two, especially if under 6 months or premature
  - malnutrition
  - diarrhoea > 5 times in 24 hours
  - vomiting > 2 times in 24 hours
  - frail or elderly
- fasting is not recommended. A normal diet should be resumed as soon as symptoms permit. Warn about the gastro-colic reflex
- babies should continue normal feeds
- avoid NSAIDs (gastric irritants)
- take paracetamol if needed for stomach cramps
- probiotics such as *Lactobacillus acidophilus* may be helpful, especially in diarrhoea following broad-spectrum antibiotics. These can be found in bio-yogurt products such as Yakult or Actimel, or (probably more effectively) in capsule form. (Although there is evidence that probiotics are effective, they were not recommended by NICE because of inconsistent results)
- loperamide may be taken by adults if diarrhoea is disabling. Avoid if there is fever, blood in the stool or severe malaise. 'The body has evolved for our survival, and not for our comfort'
- worsening advice, symptoms of dehydration

Lactose intolerance

Occasionally, after a bout of gastro-enteritis, small children may develop a temporary inability to digest lactose, which may delay the resolution of their diarrhoea. If this is suspected, suggest using lactose-free milk (e.g. SMA LF) and a lactose-free diet for up to 6 weeks.

Prescription (none for most patients)
- oral rehydration salts (see 'Self-care', page 95)
- adult patients who are at risk of dehydration, or need to take important oral medication, could be offered buccal prochlorperazine (available OTC) to stop vomiting

Action
- advise about medication, e.g. COC
- consider stopping PPI, which reduces the natural defences against GI infection
- if patient at risk of dehydration or BP low, advise temporarily stopping:
  — metformin
  — methotrexate
  — ACEI
  — diuretic
- notify HPU immediately, and inform patient, if:
  — food poisoning suspected because of history
  — blood or pus in stool
  — bacterial or protozoal infection confirmed by culture

Refer to doctor
- urgently if:
  — dehydration or severe illness
  — immunosuppressed
  — diabetes (unless you are confident in managing this)
  — bowel disease (e.g. ulcerative colitis, Crohn's disease, diverticular disease)
  — green, red or brown vomit
  — significant blood (red or black) in stools
  — possibility of ectopic pregnancy
  — abdominal tenderness or distension
  — symptoms are side-effects of a drug which will need to be changed (urgency of referral depends on why the drug was prescribed)

Cautions
- spurious or 'overflow' diarrhoea may be caused by severe constipation. If in doubt, do a rectal examination
- diarrhoea and vomiting may be an early feature of septicaemia, pyelonephritis, or ectopic pregnancy

References

Health Protection Agency. *Infectious Diarrhoea. The role of microbiological examination of faeces: quick reference guide for primary care.* London: Health Protection Agency; 2007. Available at: www.hpa.org.uk

Masukume G. Nausea, vomiting and deaths from ectopic pregnancy [letter]. *BMJ.* 2011; **343**: 163–214.

National Institute for Health and Clinical Excellence. *Diarrhoea and Vomiting in Children under 5: NICE guideline 84.* London: NIHCE; 2009. www.nice.org.uk/guidance/CG84

Passariello G, Manguso F, Guarino A, *et al*. Probiotics for treatment of acute diarrhoea in children: randomised clinical trial of five different preparations. *BMJ.* 2007; **335**: 340–6.

World Gastroenterology Organisation. *Acute Diarrhea.* Milwaukee, WI: World Gastroenterology Organisation; 2008. Available at: www.worldgastroenterology.org

Constipation

History
- duration; habitual
- how often bowels open
- consistency of motion/straining
- blood in stool, on toilet paper or in toilet pan
- abdominal pain
- vomiting
- previous abdominal operations
- unintentional weight loss
- medication (e.g. analgesics containing codeine, tricyclic antidepressants)
- diet, fluid intake, amount of exercise

Examination
- palpate abdomen
- consider rectal examination if diagnosis/severity in doubt

Self-care
- high-fibre diet. Increase intake of whole grains, apricots, prunes and dried fruit
- try Beverley-Travis natural laxative mixture: take one cup each of raisins, pitted prunes, prune concentrate, dried figs, dates and currants. Combine contents together in grinder or blender to a thickened consistency. Store in refrigerator. Dose: 2 tablespoons twice a day. Increase or decrease dose according to consistency and frequency of bowel movements
- adequate fluid intake (2 litres per day)
- increase exercise
- if stools are soft but still difficult to pass, add senna
- treatment may need to continue for several weeks
- glycerol suppositories give fast relief if there is faecal loading

Action

- review drugs, especially codeine preparations
- in adults:
  — Fybogel (ispaghula husk) may be used, if fibre intake is insufficient. Ensure adequate fluid intake
  — if stools remain hard, change to Movicol
  — if stools are still soft but hard to pass, add stimulant, e.g. senna
- in children, do not use dietary measures alone. Prescribe Movicol. See NICE guideline for more information

Refer to doctor

- urgently if:
  — associated with vomiting and/or previous abdominal surgery
  — mass or distension in abdomen
  — unexplained weight loss
  — iron-deficiency anaemia
- routinely if:
  — persistent rectal bleeding without anal symptoms
  — narrowing of stool calibre
  — in child, symptoms from first few weeks of life
  — severe, persistent constipation

References

Hale EM, Smith E, St James J, *et al.* Pilot study of the feasibility and effectiveness of a natural laxative mixture. *Geriatr Nurs.* 2007; **28**(2): 104–11.

Prodigy. *Clinical topic: Constipation.* 2011. Available at: http://prodigy.clarity.co.uk/constipation (accessed 29 August 2011).

National Institute for Health and Clinical Excellence. *Constipation in Children and Young People: NICE guideline 57.* London: NIHCE; 2010. www.nice.org.uk/guidance/CG99

Rectal problems

Haemorrhoids ('piles')
These are distended venous cushions inside the anal canal, which have a similar appearance to varicose veins. They may prolapse ('come down') on straining, when they may be visible as soft, purple grape-like swellings protruding from the anus. They may cause bleeding, itching or discomfort.

Thrombosed external pile
This is caused by a sudden leakage of blood from a small blood vessel near the anus. The blood stretches the sensitive skin and is very painful. It will gradually disperse, but if the patient presents early it is possible to incise it and relieve pain by releasing the blood clot.

Anal fissure
A split in the anal skin, thought to be caused by passing a large, hard stool. This is a common cause of pain and bleeding on defaecation. Most will heal within 6 weeks, provided that the stools remain soft.

History
- bleeding on defaecation:
  — how much, in toilet pan/on paper only
  — bright red/dark red
- pain on defaecation
- itch (suspect threadworms)
- swelling near anus, or does a swelling appear on straining
- constipation

Examination
- may be normal if haemorrhoids are internal
- any visible swelling
- any split in perianal skin
- worms may be seen

Self-care
- avoid straining
- high-fibre diet
- drink 2 litres of fluid daily
- use moist wipes, then pat area dry
- if the pain of thrombosed piles is severe, relief may be obtained by sitting on something cold

- consider Fybogel short term
- Anusol ointment and/or suppositories

Action
- prescribe Xyloproct if pain is severe

Refer to doctor
- urgently if:
  — severe bleeding or pain
  — dark blood (may come from a carcinoma high inside the bowel)
- routinely if:
  — persistent or recurrent problems

Cautions
- remember the possibility of sexual abuse or sexually transmitted diseases
- threadworms are the commonest cause of anal discomfort in children

Threadworms (pinworms)

History
- children most commonly affected
- perianal irritation
- anal pain at night
- sometimes vaginal itching
- worms may be seen – like white cotton threads – on skin or in stool

Examination
- examine the affected area for worms/trauma

Test
- tests are not necessary unless the diagnosis is in doubt
- your microbiology laboratory may supply a 'pinworm kit' containing a sticky slide
- this should be applied to the anus first thing in the morning to pick up the eggs

Self-care
- an appointment is not necessary if the parent is sure of the diagnosis
- explain that adult threadworms live for only 6 weeks – their eggs must be transferred to the mouth and swallowed for the infection to continue
- hygienic measures are necessary:
  — wash hands and scrub nails before each meal and after going to the toilet
  — bathe or shower in early morning to remove eggs laid during the night
  — don't eat food in the bedroom
  — wear close-fitting pants in bed
  — change and launder bed linen, underwear and nightclothes frequently

— vacuum bedroom carpet frequently
— cut fingernails short
— don't put fingers in the mouth
— no need to exclude from school/day care

Treatment
- mebendazole for adults (unless pregnant or breastfeeding) and children over 2 years. A second dose may be needed 2 weeks later
- piperazine/senna for children under 2 years
- treat all members of household simultaneously
- if pregnant or breastfeeding, hygiene methods alone should be used

Reference
Prodigy. *Clinical topic: Threadworm.* 2011. Available at: http://prodigy.clarity.co.uk/threadworm (accessed 29 August 2011).

Cystitis (lower urinary tract infection)

History
- duration
- dysuria
- suprapubic pain
- urgency
- frequency and nocturia
- in men, symptoms of urinary obstruction: hesitancy, straining, poor stream
- cloudy, red-brown or offensive urine
- incontinence/bedwetting
- fever (indicates pyelonephritis, *see* page 104)
- vaginal discharge
- recurrent symptoms
- sexual history
- symptoms associated with intercourse
- possibility of pregnancy
- previous history of kidney disease

Examination
- temperature
- check loins for tenderness
- examine abdomen in children and men, or if pyelonephritis suspected
- in menopausal woman with recurrent symptoms, offer examination for atrophic vaginitis
- in small boys, check the penis for redness (*see* 'Balanitis', page 105)

Tests

- urinalysis and MSU *before starting treatment* in:
  - children. Clean catch is best – providing a sterile gallipot may help. Bag or pad samples may be needed in infants. Older children should be encouraged to pass a sample directly into a sterile container, but if this proves impossible, it is reasonable to collect a sample from a container lined with clingfilm. For young girls who can use a toilet, it may make it easier to collect the sample if they sit facing the cistern
  - immunosuppressed
  - men
  - pregnant women
  - recurrent infections
  - treatment failures
- in 'simple cystitis' (lower UTI in a non-pregnant, low-risk adult woman) consider urinalysis for blood/leucocyte esterase/nitrite only if the diagnosis of lower UTI is in doubt. A positive nitrite test is 90% diagnostic of infection, but a negative result for all three indicators does not exclude infection
- arrange follow-up MSU after treatment in:
  - pregnant women
  - recurrent infections
- consider chlamydia test if suggested by sexual history, a change in vaginal discharge, pain or bleeding during or after sexual intercourse
- if associated vaginal discharge, offer speculum examination, high vaginal and cervical swabs for culture

Self-care

- adequate fluid intake
- excessive fluid intake may increase the amount of dysuria in 24 hours
- OTC remedies such as Cymalon are not recommended
- cranberry extract does not reduce the severity or duration of an episode, although it may be helpful in reducing the frequency of recurrent infections. It should not be taken by patients on anticoagulants
- if cystitis occurs after sexual intercourse, advise emptying bladder immediately afterwards

Action

- offer antibiotics for all except minor urinary infections
- in children and pregnant women, test and treat; do not wait for the MSU result before starting antibiotics. (UTI in early pregnancy increases the risk of miscarriage)
- simple cystitis in a non-pregnant woman:
  - without antibiotics, resolves in 4–9 days
  - with antibiotics, resolves in 3–8 days
  - on average, antibiotics shorten duration by 1 day
- review children and pregnant women by phone when MSU result available

Antibiotic choice

- for treating before the MSU result is known, depends on local sensitivities. Consult local guidelines or ask your microbiologist about local resistance pattern. If trimethoprim has high levels of resistance locally, ask about suitable alternatives
  — simple cystitis in a non-pregnant woman:
    – nitrofurantoin MR for 3 days
    – or trimethoprim for 3 days (depending on local patterns of antibiotic resistance)
  — pregnant woman: nitrofurantoin MR for 7 days (unless near term, in which case give cefalexin 500 mg twice daily)
  — men: trimethoprim or co-amoxiclav for 14 days (50% of men with lower UTI have prostatic involvement, and nitrofurantoin does not penetrate the prostate)
  — children: trimethoprim for 3 days (or cefalexin for 3 days if allergic to trimethoprim)
  — if MSU shows that the organism is resistant to the antibiotic prescribed, check with patient whether their symptoms have resolved. Laboratory sensitivity data do not necessarily reflect what happens to the patient
  — do not use amoxicillin for UTI unless you have an MSU showing that the organism is sensitive (50% are resistant)

Refer to doctor

- urgently if:
  — history of renal disease
  — child under 6 months
  — child, man or pregnant woman not responding to antibiotics after 48 hours
  — palpable bladder
- routinely (when UTI confirmed by MSU result) if:
  — child:
    – with organism other than *E. coli*
    – with recurrent UTI (three or more episodes)
  — man with symptoms of urinary obstruction: hesitancy, straining, poor stream
  — severe/persistent/recurrent symptoms

Cautions

- if any suspicion of pyelonephritis, *see* page 104
- women sometimes confuse the symptoms of thrush and cystitis
- chlamydia infections may cause dysuria

References

Falagas ME, Kotsantis IK, Vouloumanou EK, *et al*. Antibiotics versus placebo in the treatment of women with uncomplicated cystitis: a meta-analysis of randomized controlled trials. *J Infect*. 2009; 58(2): 91–102.

National Collaborating Centre for Women's and Children's Health. *Urinary Tract Infection in Children: diagnosis, treatment and long-term management. NICE guideline 54*. London: NIHCE; 2007. www.nice.org.uk/guidance/CG57

National Prescribing Centre. *Managing Simple UTI: don't routinely send urine for cultures, consider delayed antibiotics*. 2010. Available at: www.npci.org.uk

Perrotta C, Aznar M, Mejia R, *et al*. Oestrogens for preventing recurrent urinary tract infection in postmenopausal women. *Cochrane Database Syst Rev.* 2008; **2**: CD005131.

Richards D, Toop L, Chambers S, *et al*. Response to antibiotics of women with symptoms of urinary tract infection but negative dipstick urine test results: double blind randomised controlled trial. *BMJ.* 2005; **331**(7509): 143.

Scottish Intercollegiate Guidelines Network (SIGN). *Management of Suspected Bacterial Urinary Tract Infection in Adults: SIGN guideline 88*. Edinburgh: Scottish Intercollegiate Guidelines Network; 2006. www.sign.ac.uk/pdf/sign88.pdf

Pyelonephritis (upper urinary tract infection)

History
- fever/rigors/abdominal pain/loin pain/vomiting/confusion
- in babies, fever/vomiting/irritability/poor feeding/
- incontinence/bedwetting
- maybe symptoms of cystitis (*see* page 101)

Examination
- temperature
- pulse and blood pressure in adults
- CRT in children
- check loins for tenderness
- examine abdomen for palpable bladder

Tests
- urinalysis for blood/leucocyte esterase/nitrite
- MSU before starting treatment
- arrange follow-up MSU after treatment

Self-care
- adequate fluid intake
- analgesia – paracetamol or ibuprofen
- worsening advice

Action
- consider hospital admission or referral (see next page)
- prescribe antibiotics
- review when MSU result available

Antibiotic choice in adults (depends on local sensitivities):
- ciprofloxacin 500 mg twice daily for 7 days
- co-amoxiclav in maximum dose: 500/125 mg three times a day for 14 days is an alternative
- if pregnant, cefalexin 500 mg twice daily for 14 days

Refer to doctor
- urgently if:
  — seriously ill (dehydrated, low BP, rapid pulse)
  — immunosuppressed
  — diabetes
  — renal disease
  — pregnant
  — child
  — palpable bladder
- routinely, for investigations, if:
  — male
  — recurrent infection
  — MSU reports *Proteus* infection

 Caution
- pyelonephritis is not a minor illness, and should only be managed by experienced clinicians

Balanitis (sore penis)

History
- duration
- swelling of foreskin
- discharge
- itch
- odour
- dysuria
- previous episodes
- diabetes
- immunosuppressed
- in adults, sexual history

Examination
- gently attempt to retract foreskin in boys aged 3 and over
- assess hygiene
- localised redness/generalised cellulitis

Tests
- consider taking a swab
- send MSU for culture if no redness visible
- consider testing urine for glucose in adults

Self-care
- advise gentle cleaning with lukewarm water
- avoid soaps and detergents
- pull back foreskin for cleaning only if easily retractile, in boys aged 3 and over (ensure it is pulled down afterwards)
- if difficulty in passing urine because of pain, sit in bath

Prescription
- clotrimazole/hydrocortisone cream for mild inflammation
- flucloxacillin for 7 days if cellulitis present in a child (clarithromycin if allergic to penicillin)

Refer to doctor (?genitourinary clinic)
- urgently, if:
  — immunosuppressed
  — severe symptoms
- routinely, if:
  — recurrent episodes in children (may need surgical treatment)

Cautions
- if no visible redness, this may be a UTI
- candida is the commonest cause of balanitis in adults
- this may be the first presentation of diabetes
- very little research is available to guide practice on balanitis in children

Reference
Prodigy. *Clinical topic: Balanitis*. 2011. Available at: http://prodigy.clarity.co.uk/balanitis (accessed 29 August 2011).

8

Women's health

- Vaginal discharge
- Heavy menstrual bleeding
- Intermenstrual bleeding
- Missed pills
- Diarrhoea and vomiting on oral contraceptives
- Antibiotics and oral contraceptives
- Emergency contraception
- Mastitis
- Nipple pain

Taking a sexual history

- establish rapport first
- explain that you need to ask some sensitive questions in order to establish what is wrong
- partner gender, last sexual intercourse, sites of exposure, condom use
- previous sexual partner
- previous sexually transmitted infection (STI)
- last menstrual period (LMP), contraceptive history
- establish competency/child protection concerns (if age < 16 years)

For more information, see the British Association for Sexual Health and HIV guideline: www.bashh.org/documents/84/84.pdf (accessed 4 July 2011).

Vaginal discharge

History

- duration
- colour
- smell
- itch
- post-coital or intermenstrual bleeding
- pelvic pain
- sexual history
- dyspareunia
- possibility of pregnancy
- recent gynaecological procedure or childbirth

Examination

- a digital vaginal and speculum examination is always needed if:
  - suspected pelvic inflammatory disease, recent gynaecological procedure or childbirth (but should also have bimanual examination by a doctor, ideally same day at genito-urinary medicine clinic)
  - high risk of STI: aged < 25 or new sexual partner in the last 12 months
  - immunosuppressed
  - recurrent symptoms
  - pregnant

Tests

- take high vaginal swab
- consider also taking cervical swabs for bacterial and chlamydial tests if:
  - at increased risk of STI
  - cervicitis on examination
  - poor response to initial treatment
  - recurrent vaginal discharge
  - discharge of uncertain cause
  - after gynaecological procedure or childbirth

 Cautions

- genital herpes:
  - blisters
  - pain rather than itch
- pelvic inflammatory disease:
  - pelvic pain
  - fever
  - irregular bleeding

The two commonest causes of vaginal discharge are candida and bacterial vaginosis.

Candida

Thirty per cent of women have candida as a commensal in their vagina (i.e. it causes no symptoms).

History
- duration
- colour – usually white
- smell – may be described as yeast-like
- itch
- dyspareunia
- previous episodes
- timing with menstrual cycle
- recent broad-spectrum antibiotics
- diabetes – if so, how well controlled
- immunosuppressed
- possibility of pregnancy
- treatments already tried

Examination
- inflamed vulva, maybe fissures
- speculum examination shows white 'cottage cheese' discharge on cervix and in vagina

Tests
- if first or atypical presentation, take high vaginal swab (HVS)
- if resistant to treatment, ask laboratory to test for non-albicans *Candida* species
- if recurrent or severe symptoms, arrange FBG, FBC and ferritin

Self-care
- avoid irritating the area with soap, shower gel or bath additives
- avoid tight-fitting synthetic fabrics
- buy a clotrimazole pessary or oral fluconazole capsule (these are equally effective, although clotrimazole may give more rapid relief. The price is similar, although variable; supermarkets usually offer the lowest prices)
- clotrimazole cream (used in addition, not as an alternative) will probably relieve external itching more quickly. This can be bought more cheaply in a combination pack (which would entail two prescription charges)
- consider clotrimazole/hydrocortisone cream instead, if itching severe
- caution – clotrimazole affects latex condoms
- no need to treat sexual partner, unless they have symptoms
- no evidence to support the use of live yogurt or probiotics, although they do no harm

> ### Vaginal thrush – treatment options
>
> C200 = clotrimazole 200 mg pessaries, one at night
> C500 = clotrimazole 500 mg pessaries, one at night
> F50[2] = fluconazole 50 mg capsules, two daily
> F150 = fluconazole 150 mg capsules, one dose

Prescription

- for uncomplicated infections, give single dose C500 or F150, according to patient's preference
- if treatment failure, first try alternative above. If both have failed, give:
  — F50[2] for 7 days, *or*
  — C200 for 6 nights
- if severe or persistent symptoms, give:
  — F150 repeated after 3 days, *or*
  — C500 repeated after 3 days
- if poorly controlled diabetes or immunosuppression, give:
  — F50[2] for 7 days, *or*
  — C200 for 6 nights
- if pregnant, give:
  — C200 for 7 nights. The patient may prefer to insert the pessary manually

Refer to doctor

- routinely if:
  — recurrent symptoms. The diagnosis will be reconsidered. A supply of treatment may be given to treat recurrences as soon as they arise, or maintenance treatment may be offered for 6 months, e.g.:
    – clotrimazole 500 mg pessaries once a week
    – fluconazole 150 mg capsules once a week
    – itraconazole 200 mg capsules twice daily for 1 day, once a month

References

Nurbhai M, Grimshaw J, Watson M, *et al*. Oral versus intra-vaginal imidazole and triazole anti-fungal treatment of uncomplicated vulvovaginal candidiasis (thrush) *Cochrane Database Syst Rev*. 2007; **4**: CD002845.

British Association for Sexual Health and HIV (BASHH). *National Guideline on the Management of Vulvovaginal Candidiasis*. 2007. Available at: www.bashh.org/documents/50/50.pdf (accessed 3 August 11).

Bacterial vaginosis (BV)

Fifty per cent of women with BV are asymptomatic. It may coexist with other infections, notably candida. BV has been linked with complications of pregnancy, but this is controversial.

History
- duration
- nature of discharge – usually thin and white
- smell – may be described as fishy
- no itching or soreness
- previous episodes
- possibility of pregnancy
- treatments already tried

Examination
- speculum examination shows thin smooth white discharge coating vagina, no inflammation

Tests
- if first, recurrent or atypical presentation, or pregnancy, take high vaginal swab (HVS)
- pH testing is useful, if available. The vaginal pH is above 4.5 in this condition
- if pregnant, repeat test 1 month after treatment

Self-care
- not a sexually transmitted infection
- avoid douching
- no need to treat sexual partner
- no need to retest after treatment (unless pregnant)

Prescription
- metronidazole tabs 400 mg twice daily for 7 days. A single dose of 2 g may be used, but relapse rates are higher, *or*
- metronidazole vaginal gel 0.75% for 5 nights (40 g) *or*
- clindamycin vaginal cream for 7 nights (40 g). Caution – affects latex condoms

Reference

British Association for Sexual Health and HIV (BASHH). *National Guideline for the Management of Bacterial Vaginosis*. 2006. Available at: www.bashh.org/documents/62/62.pdf (accessed 10 March 2011).

Heavy menstrual bleeding

History
- duration and heaviness of this period
- usual pattern of menstrual cycle
- intermenstrual or post-coital bleeding (*see* page 113)
- clots/flooding
- dysmenorrhoea
- whether intrauterine contraceptive device (IUCD) or implant fitted

- need for contraception
- was this period late (possibility of miscarriage)
- hot flushes/sweats (if aged over 40)

Examination
- not necessary urgently

Tests
- FBC and ferritin

Self-care
- there is no link between passing 'clots' in the menstrual flow and internal thrombosis
- ibuprofen often significantly reduces menstrual flow. It is chemically related to mefenamic acid (Ponstan) but has a better side-effect profile. Stronger NSAIDs such as diclofenac and naproxen are now available OTC
- tranexamic acid is also usually effective
- iron supplements may be needed if loss has been heavy
- there are several options for treatment; NICE produce a useful leaflet (*see* References). The intrauterine system (IUS) is often the best choice

Prescription
- naproxen can be used as an alternative to ibuprofen
- if the above treatment fails, norethisterone will stop the bleeding within 2 days. A light period will occur after the 10-day course

Refer to doctor
- always, for vaginal examination and discussion of treatment options, once bleeding has stopped
- bleeding after 1 year of amenorrhoea (post-menopausal bleeding) should be investigated

References

National Collaborating Centre for Women's and Children's Health. *Heavy Menstrual Bleeding: Full guideline 44*. London; Royal College of Obstetricians and Gynaecologists; 2007. www. nice.org.uk/guidance/CG44

National Institute for Health and Clinical Excellence. *Heavy Menstrual Bleeding: understanding NICE guidance. NICE guideline 44*. London: NIHCE; 2007. www.nice.org.uk/guidance/CG44

Intermenstrual bleeding

History

- menstrual cycle
- date of last menstrual period (LMP)
- previous episodes
- fever
- abdominal pain
- offensive discharge
- sexual history
- first experience of penetrative sex
- any possibility of pregnancy
- contraceptive method (if on oral contraceptive, missed pills/vomiting/antibiotics)
- taking hormone replacement therapy (HRT)

Examination

- not necessary while still bleeding unless pain/fever/discharge present, in which case refer

Tests

- swab for chlamydia, take other swabs if indicated
- consider pregnancy test

Action

- if missed contraceptive pills/vomiting/antibiotic: *see* 'Missed pills' below
- if first experience of penetrative sex, reassure that some bleeding is common
- if missed HRT tablets, resume tablet taking and make appointment if bleeding persists
- otherwise, make appointment with doctor for vaginal examination when bleeding stops

Refer to doctor

- immediately if:
  — abdominal pain/fever/offensive discharge (could be pelvic inflammatory disease)
  — pregnant (may need obstetric referral)
- routinely if:
  — no obvious cause for symptom (rarely, carcinoma of cervix/uterus/ovary may present in this way)

Missed pills

Missed COCs

- missed pills are those which are more than 24 hours late (12 hours for Qlaira). When active COC pills have been missed, take the last missed pill as soon as possible and then continue as usual. This might entail taking two pills at the same time
- if less than seven pills are left in the pack, finish the active pills in the current pack and then immediately start a new pack (omitting the pill-free interval or discarding any inactive tablets)

- if inactive pills are missed in week 4 of an everyday (ED) COC, throw away the missed pills and continue as usual
- if one active pill is missed, there is no need to take additional precautions. Consider emergency contraception (EC) if pills have been missed earlier in the packet or in the last week of the previous packet
- if two or more active pills are missed in the first week, advise condoms or abstinence for 7 days (9 days for Qlaira) and consider EC if unprotected sexual intercourse (UPSI) occurred in pill-free interval or first week of pill taking

Missed POPs

- if more than 12 hours late in taking Cerazette or more than 3 hours late in taking any other POP, contraceptive cover will be lost
- advise her to take the next POP as soon as possible and continue taking the pills daily. This may entail taking two pills at the same time
- advise additional contraceptive protection for the next 48 hours and consider emergency contraception

Reference

Faculty of Sexual and Reproductive Healthcare Clinical Effectiveness Unit. *Missed Pill Recommendations*. 2011. Available at: www.fsrh.org/pdfs/CEUStatementMissedPills.pdf (accessed 15 November 2011).

Diarrhoea and vomiting on oral contraceptives

Vomiting and persistent, severe diarrhoea can interfere with the absorption of combined oral contraceptives. If vomiting occurs within 2 hours of taking any oral contraceptive, another pill should be taken as soon as possible. If the replacement pill cannot be kept down, then extra precautions will be needed (*see* Table 8.1).

With COCs, if the vomiting and diarrhoea occurs during the last seven tablets, the next pill-free interval should be omitted (in the case of ED tablets the inactive ones should be omitted).

In cases of persistent vomiting or very severe diarrhoea, additional precautions should be used during illness and also after recovery (*see* Table 8.1).

TABLE 8.1 Need for extra precautions with different types of oral contraceptives. Derived from information in *British National Formulary 61*, 2011

Type of oral contraceptive	Brand	Replacement pill not taken & retained within	Continue extra precautions after recovery for
COC	Qlaira	12 h	9 days
	Others	24 h	7 days
POP	Cerazette	12 h	2 days
	Others	3 h	2 days

Antibiotics and oral contraceptives

In *BNF 61* (March 2011), a review of the evidence for an interaction between antibiotics and contraceptives concluded that: 'No additional contraceptive precautions are required when combined oral contraceptives are used with antibacterials that do not induce liver enzymes, unless (*persistent severe*) diarrhoea or vomiting occur.' The same advice applies to progestogen-only methods. The antibiotics we recommend for the treatment of minor illness do not induce liver enzymes, so extra contraceptive precautions will no longer be necessary.

Emergency contraception (EC)

History
- if under 16, check if Fraser competent (previously Gillick competent – *see* page 116)
- date of LMP
- time since UPSI
- sexual history
- risk of sexually transmitted infection (by definition if EC is needed, the woman is at risk of an STI)
- risk of having had non-consensual sexual intercourse
- previous UPSI this cycle (may render treatment ineffective – consider copper IUCD)
- usual contraceptive method: missed pills, late injection
- previous emergency contraception this cycle
- on enzyme-inducing medication, e.g. carbamazepine, phenytoin, rifampicin
- taking St John's Wort
- breastfeeding
- past history of porphyria or asthma
- need for future contraception

Self-care
- an emergency IUCD is the most reliable option. On average, if 1000 women have UPSI, 80 will become pregnant. After taking levonorgestrel or ulipristal, 10 women will still become pregnant, but after emergency copper IUCD insertion only one
- many pharmacies provide emergency hormonal contraception free of charge. This service is usually just for under 25s, but can vary depending on local NHS policy and may depend on which pharmacist is on duty
- oral EC may cause nausea. Seek help if vomiting within 2 hours of taking levonorgestrel or 3 hours of taking ulipristal
- use condoms, or do not have penetrative sex, until next period, which may be early or late
- pregnancy test is recommended if next period more than 1 week late
- no known adverse effect on fetus if pregnancy occurs, but ectopic pregnancy more likely
- consider long-term contraception, STI screening and safe sex

Prescription (if IUCD fit declined)

- if within 72 hours of UPSI, one levonorgestrel 1.5 mg tablet
- if between 72 and 120 hours after UPSI, one ulipristal acetate 30 mg tablet
- for those on enzyme-inducing drugs, two tablets of levonorgestrel 1.5 mg, to be taken together

Refer to doctor

- if more than 120 hours since UPSI (ulipristal still has some benefit, but not licensed)
- if pregnant

Caution

- if patient vomits within 2 hours of taking levonorgestrel or 3 hours of taking ulipristal, give replacement prescription, plus domperidone tablets to be taken 30 minutes before EC dose
- if the problem is complex, you or the patient can ring the FPA helpline for advice on 0845 310 1334

References

Glasier AF, Cameron ST, Fine PM, *et al.* Ulipristal acetate versus levongestrel for emergency contraception: a randomised non-inferiority trial and meta-analysis. *Lancet.* 2010; **375**(9714): 555–62.

Prodigy. *Clinical topic: Contraception – emergency.* 2011. Available at: http://prodigy.clarity.co.uk/contraception_emergency (accessed 29 August 2011).

Legal issues around providing emergency contraception to those under 16

The legal age of consent to sexual activity is 16 in Scotland, England and Wales, and 17 in Northern Ireland. Sexual activity under the age of consent is an offence even if consensual. Offences are considered more serious (statutory rape) when the person is less than 13 years old. In England and Wales, it is legal to provide contraceptive advice and treatment to young people without parental consent, provided that the practitioner is satisfied that the Fraser criteria for competence are met:

- the young person understands the practitioner's advice
- the young person cannot be persuaded to inform their parents, or will not allow the practitioner to inform the parents, that contraceptive advice has been sought
- the young person is likely to begin or to continue having intercourse with or without contraceptive treatment
- unless she receives contraceptive advice or treatment, the young person's physical or mental health (or both) are likely to suffer

- the young person's best interest requires the practitioner to give contraceptive advice or treatment (or both) without parental consent

All available methods of emergency contraception should be offered, regardless of age, as the risk of an unwanted pregnancy outweighs that of the contraceptive.

Note: *child protection issues should be taken into account* – it is important to be satisfied that sex has been consensual and is not occurring in an incestuous relationship. If it is suspected that force has been used or that any sexual abuse has occurred, you have a duty to follow national and local child protection procedures.

References

Faculty of Sexual & Reproductive Healthcare. *Contraceptive Choices for Young People: clinical guidance.* 2010. Available at: www.fsrh.org/pdfs/ceuGuidanceYoungPeople2010.pdf (accessed 14 August 2011).

Prodigy. *Clinical topic: Contraception – emergency.* 2011. Available at: http://prodigy.clarity.co.uk/contraception_emergency (accessed 29 August 2011).

Mastitis

In lactating women, blocked milk flow is the main cause of mastitis. Milk leaks into the surrounding tissues, where molecules called cytokines cause inflammation. If milk products pass into the bloodstream, they will produce malaise and fever, even if there is no infection. Without effective milk drainage, staphylococcal infection is likely to develop.

In non-lactating women, smokers and people with diabetes are at highest risk and the bacteria responsible are different. There is no good research to guide practice in the prescription of antibiotics in this situation.

History
- lactating
- smoking
- diabetes
- fever
- location of pain
- redness of breast

Examination
- temperature
- record area of redness

- examine nipples for inflammation
- check for any suggestion of an abscess (red fluctuant lump)

Self-care
- if lactating:
  — see a breastfeeding advisor
  — continue to breastfeed from both sides, offering the affected side first
  — express any remaining milk
- paracetamol or ibuprofen to relieve pain
- warm compress, warm bath or shower
- rest
- do not wear a bra at night
- seek further advice if worsening or not improving after 48 hours

Tests
- breast-milk culture if severe, recurrent, or no response to 48 hours of antibiotics

Antibiotics for mastitis

Prescribe an antibiotic if:
- severe symptoms
- immunosuppressed or diabetes
- yellow discharge from nipple
- not improving after 12–24 hours despite effective milk removal (consider a delayed prescription)

Antibiotic choice
- in lactation:
  — flucloxacillin for 14 days
  — erythromycin if the patient is allergic to penicillin
- if not lactating:
  — co-amoxiclav for 14 days
  — erythromycin plus metronidazole if patient is allergic to penicillin

Refer to doctor
- urgently for immediate surgical referral if:
  — abscess formation suspected. Ultrasound and aspiration will be needed
  — no response after course of antibiotics (possible breast cancer)

References

Dixon JM, Khan L. Treatment of breast infection. *BMJ*. 2011; **342**: d396.

Guidelines and Audit Implementation Network (GAIN). *Guidelines on the Treatment, Management & Prevention of Mastitis*. Belfast: Guidelines and Audit Implementation Network; 2009. Available at: www.gain-ni.org/Library/Guidelines/GAIN Mastitis Guidelines.pdf (accessed 14 March 2011).

Jahanfar S, Ng CJ, Teng CL. Antibiotics for mastitis in breastfeeding women. *Cochrane Database Syst Rev*. 2009; **1**: CD005458.

Nipple pain

Pain during breastfeeding is usually due to problems with attachment of the baby to the breast.

History
- one or both sides affected
- onset in relation to childbirth
- severity, type and timing of pain
- does baby have tongue tie, oral thrush or nappy rash?
- does nipple blanch during feeds or when it is cold? If so, does it become red afterwards?
- discharge from nipple

Examination
- inverted nipples
- loss of colour in the nipples or areola
- pink or red colour, flaking, shininess, crusting
- fissure

Possible causes
- sore and fissured nipples due to friction and poor positioning (commonest)
  — problems usually start early, pain occurs during feed and may be severe
  — self-care: see breastfeeding advisor. Apply Vaseline to any broken skin
- candida
  — usually bilateral
  — delayed by a few weeks, unless woman has had recent candida infection
  — burning and itching
  — nipples appear pale, fissured or normal
  — self-care: apply miconazole 2% cream to nipples after each feed for 2 weeks, and wipe away any remaining cream before next feed
  — treat baby with oral miconazole gel (*see* page 29)
- bacterial infection
  — yellow discharge from nipple
  — persistent fissure
  — prescription: sodium fusidate ointment after each feed for 7 days. If severe, give oral flucloxacillin (or erythromycin if patient is allergic to penicillin)

- eczema
  - burning and itching
  - redness, vesicles, crusting or scaling
  - base of nipple may be unaffected
  - self-care: consider allergy to creams or new food given to baby. Avoid soap, shower gel, etc. Apply hydrocortisone or Eumovate ointment twice daily after feeds until recovered, and wipe away any remaining cream before next feed
- Raynaud's disease of nipple
  - nipple may blanch during feed or when cold, then become red
  - intermittent pain persists after feed, and may be severe
  - self-care: keep warm, avoid smoking and caffeine
  - prescription: nifedipine capsules 5 mg three times a day for two weeks. May be continued if necessary

Refer to doctor

- urgently for surgical referral if:
  - unilateral eczema not responding to treatment (could be breast cancer)

Reference

Prodigy. *Clinical topic: Breastfeeding problems*. 2011. Available at: http://prodigy.clarity.co.uk/breastfeeding_problems (accessed 29 August 2011).

9

Mental health

People who present with minor illness often have underlying mental health problems. Sometimes they will present these openly to you, but more often they will tell you about their physical symptoms because they perceive these as being more acceptable. You do not need to be an expert in mental health to pick these problems up, and it is not necessary to make a definite diagnosis in order to help; often in primary care the problems arise from relationships, work or housing issues or debt, for which you may be able to suggest appropriate local or national services. Whatever the problems, the patient's ability to cope will be improved by encouraging them to exercise (outdoors if possible) and to learn techniques which enable them to deeply relax.

Depression

This is a very common condition, in which physical symptoms are often presented initially. Be aware that it may be an underlying problem in any consultation. Any age group can be affected. The diagnosis is easily overlooked in older people. Depression in children requires specialist management.

History
- active, empathetic listening. You may be the first person to hear the patient's story
- how long has the patient felt low
- any special reason, e.g. bereavement, childbirth, relationship difficulties, financial worries, stress at work
- core symptoms: sadness, lack of interest/enjoyment. 'What are you looking forward to?'
- appetite or weight change
- sleep disturbance/fatigue
- feelings of worthlessness
- thoughts of death: 'have you ever felt that life wasn't worth living?'
- loss of concentration/poor memory
- ask: 'How will you know when you are better? What will you be doing that you aren't doing now?'
- previous episodes and treatment, and what previously helped them to resolve their problems

- medication, alcohol intake, recreational drugs
- risk factors, e.g. previous history, chronic illness, dementia

Examination
- observe body language, especially moist eyes, trembling lower lip, avoiding eye contact
- ask patient to complete a validated questionnaire: Patient Health Questionnaire 9 (PHQ-9), Hospital Anxiety and Depression Scale (HADS), or Beck Depression Inventory-II (BDI-II)

Self-care
- consider practical problem solving, e.g. change of job
- daily exercise, especially walking outdoors with relative, friend or dog, will help
- try to resume activities previously enjoyed
- consider learning/using relaxation techniques (depression is often driven by anxiety)
- if alcohol and substance misuse are part of the problem, consider contacting appropriate agencies
- ensure a regular intake of healthy food, including whole grains
- avoid excessive caffeine
- though controversial, there is some evidence that the following supplements may help:
  — omega-3 fish oils, 1g daily
  — vitamin B complex
  — vitamin D in winter

Actions
- empathise and be positive about recovery
- remind patient that they have already learnt coping strategies that have previously helped them
- recommend sleep hygiene (*see* 'Insomnia', page 123)
- if taking regular medication, check side-effects in the *British National Formulary* (*BNF*). Benzodiazepines, steroids, simvastatin, opioids like codeine, varenicline, propranolol, anticonvulsants and hormonal medications including contraceptives are some of the drugs that may precipitate depression
- if work-related stress, would time off, limited duties or reduced hours help?
- recommend self-help books and websites (*see* 'Self-care resources' page 127)
- consider referring to counsellor, or other form of talking therapy
- if severe, consider referral for antidepressants – emphasise not addictive/3-week delay before onset of action/course will last several months
- St John's Wort is not recommended by NICE because of lack of standardization of products and drug interactions. However, there is a considerable body of evidence to show that it is as effective as some SSRIs, and it avoids the perceived stigma of an antidepressant prescription. It interacts with many drugs, notably combined oral contraceptives, warfarin, amlodipine, triptans (for migraine) and anticonvulsants. See Appendix 1 of *BNF*
- if suicidal thoughts are expressed but patient declines referral, give local phone number of the Samaritans (www.samaritans.org) and discuss with doctor afterwards

Refer to doctor or community mental health team

- urgently if:
  — if symptoms are severe or suicidal thoughts are expressed

References

Appleton KM, Rogers PJ, Ness AR. Updated systematic review and meta-analysis of the effects of n-3 long-chain polyunsaturated fatty acids on depressed mood. *Am J Clin Nutr.* 2010; **91**(3): 757–70.

National Collaborating Centre for Mental Health. *Depression in Adults: NICE guideline 90.* London: NIHCE; 2009. www.nice.org.uk/guidance/CG90

Rahimi R, Nikfar S, Abdollahi M. Efficacy and tolerability of *Hypericum perforatum* in major depressive disorder in comparison with selective serotonin reuptake inhibitors: a meta-analysis. *Prog Neuro-Psychoph.* 2009; **33**(1): 118–27.

Insomnia

Insomnia is common and subjective. Some people only require 4 or 5 hours sleep a night, whereas others need 10 or more. The amount of sleep required tends to lessen with age and also with lower activity levels. A 'good' night's sleep is not the same for everyone. Almost everyone will have periods of insomnia at some stage.

History

- what is the patient's concern about the sleep pattern
- when did the problem start, and what was happening to them at that time
- what is the sleep pattern
  — difficulty getting off to sleep
  — recurrent waking during the night
  — early morning waking feeling unrefreshed
- does the patient take daytime naps
- does their partner say that they snore and are restless
- any symptoms of depression (*see* page 121)
- general health
- medication
- caffeine, nicotine, alcohol, recreational drugs
- lifestyle – e.g. shift work
- what are the patient's expectations – explore their ideas

Consider causes

- physical: pain, itching, shortness of breath, nocturia, indigestion/gastro-oesophageal reflux, tinnitus, discomfort
- physiological: shift work, jet lag, pregnancy, irregular meals, low light levels during the time awake
- psychological: emotional upsets, worries, bereavement
- psychiatric: especially depression, hypomania

- pathological: sleep apnoea, restless legs syndrome
- pharmacological: is patient on any medication possibly causing insomnia, e.g. SSRIs, bupropion, lamotrigine, propranolol, corticosteroids, salbutamol, theophylline, pseudoephedrine or laxatives, or taking excessive caffeinated drinks, alcohol, recreational drugs or nicotine
- social: new baby, shift work, enuretic child, partner who has nocturia or who snores

Examination
- look for agitation, depressed affect, 'washed out' appearance
- note if BMI > 30 (associated with sleep apnoea syndrome)

Self-care
- consider keeping a sleep diary, which can be downloaded free from http://yoursleep.aasmnet.org/pdf/sleepdiary.pdf
- try to keep to regular times for going to bed and waking up
- avoid napping during the day
- don't lie in after a poor night's sleep
- avoid caffeine, nicotine and alcohol within 6 hours of going to bed
- consider giving up caffeine altogether
- regular exercise is helpful, but not within 4 hours of bedtime
- try not to eat a heavy meal late at night
- a bedtime ritual (e.g. warm bath, milky drink) may help
- try to relax before going to bed. Relaxation exercises or training (e.g. hypnotherapy) can be helpful; also yoga, t'ai chi, meditation, reading and listening to relaxing music
- keep the bedroom quiet, dark, and at a comfortable temperature (usually cooler than other rooms)
- only use the bedroom for sleep and sex. Banish the TV
- don't keep checking the time throughout the night
- avoid lying in bed unable to get to sleep – it is better to get up and do something fairly mindless but useful, e.g. ironing
- don't drive if you feel sleepy
- over the counter remedies such as Nytol may contain sedative antihistamines (which are temporarily effective but often cause morning drowsiness) or herbs such as valerian (which has not been shown to be effective). They are not recommended
- the website http://yoursleep.aasmnet.org has useful self-care advice

Action
- If work-related stress, would time off, limited duties or reduced hours help?

Prescription/OTC
- hypnotic drugs such as temazepam may cause addiction, daytime drowsiness and rebound insomnia on stopping. They are best avoided if possible
- if essential, give temazepam 10 mg tablets, one on alternate nights for a maximum of 14 days. Warn that they may impair driving the next morning and that alcohol should be avoided when they are used. Make it clear that this is a one-off prescription

Refer to doctor
- if psychiatric problem
- if insomnia is due to prescribed drugs or treatable physical cause
- if obese and reporting snoring and excessive tiredness (may need assessment for sleep apnoea syndrome)
- if risk to safety (e.g. driving when tired)
- if problem persists for more than 4 weeks (to consider referral and/or melatonin in people over 55)

References

Prodigy. *Clinical topic: Insomnia*. 2011. Available at: http://prodigy.clarity.co.uk/insomnia (accessed 29 August 2011).

Taibi DM, Landis CA, Petry H, *et al*. A systematic review of valerian as a sleep aid: safe but not effective. *Sleep Med Rev*. 2007; **11**(3): 209–30.

Anxiety/panic attacks/phobias

History
- active, empathetic listening
- why have they come
- recent problems: at work, at home, with family or partner, financial
- previous mental health problems, and how they resolved them
- caffeine, alcohol, recreational drugs
- medication: decongestants, salbutamol, corticosteroids
- symptoms: feeling on edge or restless, dizziness, tiredness, palpitations, dry mouth, excessive sweating, weight loss, urinary frequency, sleep disturbance
- panic attacks

Examination
- observe body language, especially tremor

Tests
- take blood for thyroid function tests, if not recently done

Self-care
- consider practical problem solving, e.g. a change of job
- daily exercise, especially walking outdoors with relative, friend or dog, will help
- moderate or stop intake of caffeine, alcohol and recreational drugs
- relaxation exercises or training (e.g. hypnotherapy) can be helpful; also yoga, t'ai chi, meditation, reading and listening to relaxing music
- self-help resources (*see* page 127)

Actions

- recommend sleep hygiene (*see* 'Insomnia', page 123)
- if work-related stress, would time off, limited duties or reduced hours help?
- empathise and be positive about recovery
- if panic attacks, strongly reassure that they will not cause physical harm, such as a heart attack
- remind patient that they have already learnt coping strategies that have previously helped them
- explain limitations of drug treatment for anxiety

Refer to doctor or community mental health team

- if drug treatment requested or follow-up required

Reference

National Collaborating Centre for Mental Health. *Generalised Anxiety Disorder and Panic Disorder (with or without Agoraphobia) in Adults: NICE guideline 113*. London: NIHCE; 2011. www.nice.org.uk/guidance/CG113

Hyperventilation

History

- episodes of being 'unable to take a deep-enough breath'
- absence of other respiratory symptoms, e.g. cough/malaise
- precipitating stress
- previous episodes
- chest discomfort
- tingling round mouth, hands, feet
- spasm of hands and feet (tetany)
- agoraphobia and panic disorder (50% hyperventilate)
- asthma (up to 30% hyperventilate)

Examination (to exclude respiratory disease)

- observe respiration – often irregular or sighing, using upper chest muscles
- note the ratio of inspiration to expiration:
  — normally about 1 : 2
  — in asthma, expiration may be prolonged and through pursed lips
  — in hyperventilation, inspiration may be more energetic and expiration is not prolonged
- examine chest
  — breath sounds equal on both sides (to exclude pneumothorax)
  — no wheeze (asthma)
- record peak flow (if low, *see* 'Asthma exacerbation', page 21)

Test

- pulse oximetry, if available, may demonstrate to the patient that they are hyperventilating

Action

- explain problem. Reassure that tingling in arms and hands is not a symptom of a heart attack
- if acute, ask patient to breathe slowly in and out of paper bag, or put hands on head to splint upper chest
- show patient how to breathe using the diaphragm
- suggest yoga (breathing exercises and relaxation both likely to be helpful)
- relaxation exercises/hypnotherapy may lower the underlying emotional arousal

Refer to doctor

- urgently if:
  — unequal/abnormal breath sounds
- peak flow less than 75% of predicted value
  — problem does not respond promptly to treatment
- routinely if:
  — underlying stresses need attention
  — breathing pattern remains disturbed (may need specialist physiotherapy referral)

Reference

Patient UK. *Hyperventilation*. 2011. Available at: www.patient.co.uk/doctor/Hyperventilation.htm (accessed 24 April 2011).

Self-care resources

Books/CD-ROMs

Your local library may have a Books on Prescription scheme with recommended titles and online resources.

Griffin J, Tyrell I. *How to Lift Depression Fast*. Brighton: Human Givens; 2004. ISBN: 978-1-899398-41-6.

Griffen J, Tyrell I. *How to Master Anxiety: all you need to know to overcome stress, panic attacks, trauma, phobias, obsessions and more*. Brighton: Human Givens; 2006. ISBN: 978-1-899398-81-2.

Branch R, Willson R. *Cognitive Behavioural Therapy For Dummies*. Chichester: John Wiley & Sons; 2010. ISBN: 978-0-470-66541-1.

Johnstone M. *I Had a Black Dog*. London: Robinson; 2007. ISBN: 978-1-84529-589-9.

Skynner R, Cleese J. *Families and How to Survive Them*. London: Vermilion; 1993. ISBN: 0-7493-1410-9.

Websites:

- MoodGYM: www.moodgym.anu.edu.au. Free online cognitive behavioural therapy (CBT)
- Living Life to the Full: www.llttf.com. Free online CBT and other useful resources

- Human Givens Institute: www.hgi.org.uk. Explanation of how unmet emotional needs can cause many mental health problems

Agencies

- Relate, for relationship difficulties. www.relate.org.uk
- Drinkline – National Alcohol Helpline. 0800 917 8282
- FRANK: Friendly, confidential drugs advice. www.talktofrank.com, 0800 776 600
- Citizens' Advice Bureau (particularly helpful for debt or benefit problems)
- National Debtline – offers free, confidential and independent help over the phone for people in England, Scotland and Wales: 0800 808 4000. You can also download publications from their website: www.nationaldebtline.co.uk
- Consumer Credit Counselling Service (CCCS) – provides free and confidential counselling on debt problems, including personal budgeting and credit advice. 0800 138 1111, www.cccs.co.uk
- Community Legal Advice (CLA). If you qualify for legal aid and live in England or Wales, CLA can provide free help or legal advice over the phone about debt, housing, employment, education, welfare benefits and tax credits. 0845 345 4345, www.communitylegaladvice.org.uk
- Samaritans, a listening ear for all types of problems. 08457 909 090, www.samaritans.org
- Cruse Bereavement Care. 0844 477 9400, www.crusebereavementcare.org.uk
- National Domestic Violence Helpline (24hr): Freephone 0808 2000 247, www.national.domesticviolencehelpline.co.uk
- Expert Patients Programme, for people with long-term conditions. 0800 988 5550, www.expertpatients.co.uk
- Local counsellors (or other talking therapy)
- Health visitor (for parents of children under five)

10

Injuries

Sprains and strains

History
- severity of impact (may suggest likely consequences)
- relevant medical and drug history, particularly osteoporosis and anticoagulants
- location of any pain and what makes it worse
- timing of pain. Immediate pain and loss of function make fracture more likely, whereas delayed pain and swelling suggest soft-tissue injury
- functional loss (e.g. weakness)
- instability
- neurological symptoms

Examination
- swelling (NB: this takes time to develop – in primary care, patients often present very early)
- bruising
- deformity
- bony tenderness
- restriction of movement. If passive movements are pain-free, then fracture is unlikely
- assess circulation and sensation distal to injury

Self-care
- Follow PRICE for 3 days after the injury:
  — Protect from further injury
  — Rest: avoid activity for 3 days, but then mobilise
  — Ice (e.g. pack of frozen peas, wrapped in a towel to avoid skin damage)
  — Compression (e.g. with Tubigrip) may be a valuable early treatment for joint injuries, with the exception of the ankle where there is no evidence of benefit
  — Elevation above the level of the heart

- Avoid HARM for 3 days:
  — **H**eat (e.g. hot baths, heat pads)
  — **A**lcohol (increases bleeding and swelling)
  — **R**unning (or other exercise)
  — **M**assage (may worsen bleeding and swelling)
- take paracetamol or use topical NSAID (e.g. ketoprofen gel) for pain relief
- oral NSAIDs are *not* recommended in the first 48 hours, because they may delay the healing process. Inflammation plays an important part in healing

Refer to accident and emergency (A&E)
- urgently if:
  — child protection concerns
  — swelling of an area and known bleeding disorder (e.g. swollen knee + haemophilia)
  — inability to bear weight (walk four steps). Ankle sprains are often painful on initial walking and then improve
  — suspected dislocation, muscle tear or tendon rupture (deformity or instability)
  — suspected haemarthrosis (painful joint swelling immediately after injury)
  — suspected damage to nerves or circulation
  — wound penetrating joint
  — large intramuscular haematoma
  — suspected fracture (see box below)

Indications for X-ray after acute injury

Ankle: pain over the malleolus and one of the following:
- bone tenderness along the distal 6 cm of the posterior edge of the fibula or tip of the lateral malleolus
- bone tenderness along the distal 6 cm of the posterior edge of the tibia or tip of the medial malleolus

Foot: pain in the midfoot zone and one of the following:
- bone tenderness at base of the fifth metatarsal
- bone tenderness of the navicular bone (distal to the medial malleolus)

Knee:
- age 55 years or above
- tenderness at the head of fibula
- isolated tenderness of patella
- inability to flex knee to 90 degrees

Caution
- any injury in a non-mobile child should raise child protection concerns

References

Prodigy. *Clinical topic: Sprains and strains*. 2011. Available at: http://prodigy.clarity.co.uk/sprains_and_strains (accessed 29 August 2011).

Stovitz S, Johnson R. NSAIDs and musculoskeletal treatment. *Phys Sportsmed*. 2003; **31**(1): 35–41.

Head injury

History

- how did it happen and how long ago
- loss of consciousness
- confusion, amnesia, drowsiness, convulsions
- neurological disturbance (e.g. numbness, paralysis, double vision)
- vomiting
- headache
- neck pain
- blood or clear fluid from ear or nose
- bleeding disorder, anticoagulants
- recent intake of alcohol or recreational drug

Examination

- is the patient still confused or drowsy
- examine site of injury
- check pupils:
  — are they equal
  — do they react to light
  — photophobia

Self-care for adult

- rest as much as possible
- take paracetamol, if needed, for headache
- inform employer about head injury, if appropriate, and consider graded return to work
- until completely recovered, avoid:
  — being alone or out of telephone contact
  — alcohol or sedative medicines
  — NSAIDs (for the first 3 days)
  — contact sports
  — driving or operating machinery
  — travelling alone without a mobile phone
- go to A&E immediately if:
  — you become drowsy or confused
  — fluid leaks from your ear or nose
  — you develop problems with seeing, understanding or speaking
  — you develop loss of balance, or weakness in your arms or legs

— your headache gets worse

— you vomit again

Self-care for child

- take paracetamol if required for headache
- eat only light meals for 1 or 2 days
- until completely recovered, *avoid*:
    - leaving child alone. Check them every couple of hours while they are asleep (but do allow them to sleep, don't keep them awake)
    - giving ibuprofen
    - overexcitement
    - contact sports and rough play
- inform teacher that child has had a head injury, if appropriate, and consider graded return to school
- go to A&E immediately if child:
    - becomes drowsy or confused
    - leaks fluid leaks from ear or nose
    - develops problems with seeing, understanding or speaking
    - develops loss of balance, or weakness in arms or legs
    - complains of worsening headache
    - cries persistently
    - vomits repeatedly

Refer urgently to A&E if:

- age > 65 years
- bleeding disorder, or on anticoagulants
- previous brain surgery
- substance intoxication
- high-energy impact to head, e.g. fall from a height of > 1 m or > 5 stairs
- any history of loss of consciousness or amnesia
- confusion, convulsions or any other neurological disturbance
- vomiting (more than once in an adult or more than three times in a child)
- persistent and worsening headache
- suspicion of a non-accidental injury (e.g. child under three, inadequate explanation, delayed presentation, other injuries, previous child protection concerns)
- suspected skull fracture (periorbital haematoma without local injury, deafness, clear cerebrospinal fluid from ear or nose, bleeding from ear)
- pupils unequal or non-reactive, or photophobia
- no one to supervise patient at home

Reference

Prodigy. *Clinical topic: Head injury*. 2011. Available at: http://prodigy.clarity.co.uk/head_injury (accessed 29 August 2011).

Road traffic accident – assessment

Be aware that patients may present for a wider range of reasons than concern over symptoms; they may think it important that they attend to justify a future claim for compensation, or have been advised to be 'checked over' by the police or an insurance company.

History
- date and time of the accident
- details of the accident
- direction of impact
- if in a car, whether a seat belt was worn and whether there was a head restraint; whether passenger or driver
- whether air bags were activated
- descriptions of the injuries: pain, stiffness, bruising, etc.
- if neck pain, was it immediate with restricted movement, or delayed?
- psychological effects: shaking, insomnia, nightmares, fear of driving, flashbacks (important for compensation)
- time off work/school

Examination
- appropriate to affected area
- extent of grazing and bruising – measure these
- movement of affected limbs or neck

Action
- give treatment and advice dependent on and appropriate to the injuries
- sketch areas of grazing and bruising, or recommend a police photograph

Caution
- often the main purpose of the patient's visit is to document the injuries for a possible future compensation claim. Record the details carefully

Bites – animal and human

History
- which animal (NB: answer may not be truthful, if human bites)
- date/time of bite
- did it happen abroad
- immunosuppressed
- diabetes
- chronic liver disease
- splenectomy
- heart valve problem
- prosthetic joint

Examination
- cellulitis
- discharge
- teeth in wound

Tests
- consider wound swab

Self-care
- check for signs of infection, and if these develop, seek help immediately
- for bite on leg, elevate the leg

Action
- if fresh wound, irrigate with warm water
- consider need for vaccination against tetanus and hepatitis B
- consider post-exposure prophylaxis against rabies and HIV

Antibiotics for animal and human bites

Give antibiotics if:
- human or cat bite
- affecting the hand, foot or face
- puncture wound
- possible bone or joint penetration
- immunosuppressed
- prosthetic joint
- heart valve problem

Antibiotic choice for 7 days
- co-amoxiclav
- if allergic to penicillin, give doxycycline 100 mg twice daily plus metronidazole 400 mg three times daily

Refer urgently to A&E if
- penetrating wound affecting deeper structures
- bites to poorly vascularised areas, e.g. ear or nose
- facial wounds (unless very minor)
- suspected foreign body in wound, or in need of closure
- high-risk group: immunosuppressed, diabetes, severe liver disease, splenectomy
- child with safeguarding concerns
- wounds over or near a prosthetic joint
- risk of rabies

References

[No authors listed]. Managing bites from humans and other mammals. *Drug Ther Bull*. 2004; **42**(9): 67–71.

Health Protection Agency. *Guidelines for the Management of Human Bite Injuries: guidance for healthcare professionals on dealing with injuries where teeth break the skin*. London: Health Protection Agency; 2005. Available at: www.hpa.org.uk

Prodigy. *Clinical topic: Bites – human and animal*. 2011. Available at: http://prodigy.clarity.co.uk/bites_human_and_animal (accessed 29 August 2011).

Insect bites and stings

There is a temptation to treat too many insect bites or stings with antibiotics because the appearance of the normal inflammatory response to the sting toxin may look similar to infection. In fact, very few bites in the UK become infected. If the bite was sustained abroad, record the details in the medical records carefully in case the patient presents later with symptoms that could be a disease from the bite, such as malaria or leishmaniasis.

History
- site
- date and time of bite/sting, if known
- nature of insect, if known
- itching
- previous severe reaction to bites (suggests allergy)
- systemic symptoms (malaise, breathing difficulty, generalized rash)

Examination
- temperature
- size of reaction
- lymphangitis or cellulitis
- is sting still in situ (rare)

Self-care
- wash area with soap and water
- apply ice pack to reduce swelling
- try not to scratch – consider brushing with a clean paintbrush to reduce itching without damaging the skin
- take oral antihistamine, e.g. cetirizine
- use topical crotamiton to reduce itch
- piezoelectric devices to reduce itching (e.g. Zapperclick) are available for around £7
- if still itching, consider adding oral chlorphenamine at night, if sedation tolerated
- seek help urgently if you develop breathing difficulties or generalised rash
- after tick bites, seek help if rash or fever develops

Action

- if stinger still in place, remove it as soon as possible by scraping with a scalpel blade, not tweezers
- remove ticks as soon as possible. Specialist tick removers (e.g. Trix Tick-Lasso) are available, otherwise tweezers may be used. Heat, Vaseline and alcohol are not recommended
- severe local reactions may require oral prednisolone, 40 mg/day for adults
- it may sometimes be difficult to distinguish the expected normal inflammatory response or allergy from infection. Allergic reactions usually occur within the first 24 hours. Signs of infection usually develop after 24 hours, with increasing redness, tenderness and swelling. Other signs may include:
  - — fever
  - — pus
  - — lymphangitis (tracking)
  - — local lymph node enlargement (though this can also occur in allergy)
- if infection suspected, treat with flucloxacillin (clarithromycin if allergic to penicillin)
- if still itching after antihistamine, consider adding oral ranitidine (unlicensed indication), or if sleep is disturbed, chlorphenamine at night (if sedation acceptable)

Refer to A&E urgently if

- swelling of lips or tongue
- anaphylactic shock (extremely rare)

Refer to doctor

- routinely, for consideration of allergy clinic referral, if:
  - — local skin reaction over 10 cm in diameter

References

Karppinen A, Kautiainen H, Petman L, *et al*. Comparison of cetirizine, ebastine and loratadine in the treatment of immediate mosquito-bite allergy. *Allergy*. 2002; 57(6): 534–7.

Prodigy. *Clinical topic: Bites – insect*. 2011. Available at: http://prodigy.clarity.co.uk/insect_bites_and_stings (accessed 29 August 2011).

Sunburn

History

- country and duration of exposure
- sunscreen usage

Examination

- temperature
- extent of burn
- redness

- blistering
- skin loss

Self-care
- cool the skin by having a cool shower or bath
- drink plenty of cool fluids
- avoid alcohol and caffeine
- apply moisturising cream or aloe vera gel (only to intact skin)
- leave blisters intact if possible
- sun advice:
  — some sun exposure is beneficial – 15 minutes per day is recommended
  — avoid the sun when it is at its hottest
  — apply sunscreen regularly (at least sun protection factor 15, with ultraviolet A and B protection)
  — dress to protect your skin
- apply non-adherent dressings to areas of skin loss

Action
- if a dressing is needed, use Jelonet or Granuflex. Do not apply silver sulfadiazine

Caution
- if temperature is elevated, assess level of hydration and treat for heatstroke with rest, fluids and cooling

References
Hussain S, Ferguson C. *Silver Sulphadiazine Cream in Burns*. 2006. www.bestbets.org/bets/bet.php?id=515 (accessed 28 November 2011).

University of Texas, School of Nursing, Family Nurse Practitioner Program. *Evaluation, Management and Treatment of Sunburn in Adults*. Austin (TX): University of Texas, School of Nursing; 2007. Available at: www.guideline.gov

11

Management of minor illness

Evidence-based practice

It is helpful for all clinicians working in primary care to be consistent and evidence based in managing minor illness. Where differences in practice are apparent, you should be able to access up-to-date, high-quality research evidence to aid discussion and help you to reach agreement. Critical analysis of published research has become highly complex and very time consuming; thankfully, there are now several agencies such as the Cochrane Collaboration who analyse the evidence on your behalf, and provide easy access to this information on the Internet.

Although these reviews will explore possible flaws in the published papers, there are several factors that inherently bias the whole process of evaluating evidence. They include:
- the rigorous standards and large sample sizes now expected in clinical trials lead to very high cost, which makes it difficult to attract funding other than from pharmaceutical companies with a high turnover
- participants in research trials are usually healthy or have just the one disease requiring the treatment being researched, whereas in practice patients often have several diseases and may be taking many drugs
- trials on new drugs are too short to pick up long-term side-effects – this has to come later from monitoring
- when real outcomes are too infrequent to be examined, surrogate measures are used (e.g. serum cholesterol as opposed to death from heart attack), but these may not reflect the true outcome
- few trials examine the whole patient: an antihypertensive may reduce the risk of stroke, but did it cause more falls or road traffic accidents due to faintness?
- funded research is more likely to favour the sponsor's product
- negative results are less likely to be published
- old drugs may appear inadequately researched compared to new ones
- little research is conducted in primary care
- therapies that do not employ the same disease categories as Western medicine are almost impossible to research using randomised controlled trials
- many established therapies do not have a good evidence base because it would be

unethical to withhold them for trial purposes. No evidence of effectiveness is not the same as evidence of ineffectiveness

So what we call 'evidence' is an artificial construction, a useful concept but not to be confused with truth. Patients will have a very different perspective to clinicians on what factors would persuade them to try a new therapy. Bearing these limitations in mind, it is important to realise that guidance needs to be placed in the context of your patient's particular situation. The more experienced you become, the more you will deviate from the standard advice; it is important that your reasons are documented.

We recommend the following sources:

- Prodigy: http://prodigy.clarity.co.uk (excellent, evidence-based, practical guidance). The authors of this book contribute to Evidence Summaries, and the recommendations given here were extensively checked against Prodigy guidance at the time of writing
- NHS Evidence: www.evidence.nhs.uk (many useful resources, including the *BNF* and the Cochrane Library). An Athens password is needed in order to access some of the resources; those working in the NHS can obtain this by registering on the site
- Trip database: www.tripanswers.org for the answer to that awkward question

Holistic care

It will be apparent from reading the other chapters of this book that the previous optimism of Western medicine about the eradication of infectious diseases by antibiotics has not been fulfilled. The more that we research these drugs, the more evidence we find that their benefits in most cases of minor illness are marginal, yet little evidence exists to support alternative treatments (including traditional nursing advice about rest, fluids and regular antipyretic medicines). Nor is such evidence likely to be provided because, despite the recommendations of the Medical Research Council in 1997, funding for research into minor illness and the relief of self-limiting symptoms remains very small.

You may feel that this lack of evidence-based treatments leaves you in an awkward position: the patient is coming to you for help and you have little to offer. But your priority must be to establish that there is no serious disease, and if so to reassure the patient accordingly and give appropriate 'worsening advice'. Patients do not necessarily want advice on managing their illness. It is important to be sensitive to their beliefs and expectations, or 'agenda'. They may have attended in order to legitimise their illness to an employer, or at the insistence of a relative. Social factors, such as an impending holiday or examination, will often be of far greater importance to patients than any medical issues, and will inevitably influence their assessment of the relative risks and benefits of any treatment. Furthermore, offering unnecessary advice on treatment only encourages the patient to come back next time they have the same symptoms, which is wasteful for the health service and creates a culture of dependency for the patients.

In Western medicine, the 'placebo effect' is regarded as a nuisance which interferes with the evaluation of the 'real' effects of a treatment in clinical trials. Yet the placebo effect is itself very real, and represents the influence of the patient's belief on the intrinsic healing ability of the body. You can harness this effect very easily, by establishing a good relationship with the patient, being positive and emphasising that a good recovery is likely. The placebo effect of any treatment that you suggest will be enhanced by the fact that you have recommended it. If you recommend a treatment which does not have a good evidence base, you will need to use your clinical judgement whether to share this information with the patient (which will inevitably reduce the effectiveness). It is also clearly inappropriate to recommend such a treatment if there is a risk that it may do harm.

References

Mantzoukas S. A review of evidence-based practice, nursing research and reflection: levelling the hierarchy. *J Clin Nurs*. 2008; **17**: 214–23.

Miller FG, Colloca L, Kaptchuk TJ. The placebo effect: illness and interpersonal healing. *Perspect Biol Med*. 2009; **52**(4): 518.

Medical Research Council. *Primary Health Care: MRC topic review*. London: Medical Research Council; 1997. pp. 44–5.

Children

The examination of children requires a child-friendly environment and special skills: see the 'Spotting the sick child' link below.

- bring your face to their level
- keeping your voice soft, explain and ask permission for examination
- talk about something of interest to them
- encourage parent to cuddle them
- non-threatening examination first – e.g. hands
- then chest, before the screaming gets too loud
- with an anxious or uncooperative child, first listen to the chest through thin clothes, then undress the child and listen again
- if the child is screaming by then, listen carefully during inspiration
- leave throat until last, and only examine if necessary
- firm hold needed for ear examination
- if you need to examine the genital area, say something like 'It's OK for me to examine you because I'm a nurse, and Mummy (or Daddy) has said that it's all right'

All nurses working with children should be aware of current advice on safeguarding children, and should have undergone training to at least Level 2. This can be accessed online by NHS staff at www.corelearningunit.nhs.uk.

References

HM Government. *Working Together to Safeguard Children: a guide to inter-agency working to safeguard and promote the welfare of children*. London: TSO; 2006. Available at: www.education.gov.uk/publications
www.spottingthesickchild.com

Infections

The traditional Western explanation of the infectious process portrays the human body as a sterile environment which has been invaded by a hostile organism. Our scientists' efforts have been concentrated on finding newer and better chemical weapons to defeat these enemy forces. However, the spread of antibiotic resistance is causing increasing concern. Our ability to develop new antibiotics is limited; all of the antibiotics in our formulary were developed more than 30 years ago.

We are beginning to see that this warlike model is fundamentally flawed. The human body is more like an ecosystem, supporting a myriad of other organisms far greater in number than the cells in our body. Some of them are essential for our survival, like the intestinal bacteria that manufacture vitamin K. Broad-spectrum antibiotics dramatically alter our internal flora, leading to side-effects such as diarrhoea and vaginal thrush.

Many of the organisms that can cause infections are normal inhabitants of the healthy human body (commensals). The process which causes them to become pathogenic is not well understood, but often seems to be initiated by a fall in the vigilance of the immune system rather than a change in the organism itself. The immune system has intricate links with all other systems of the body, and is susceptible to the effects of nutrition and psychosocial stress. It follows from this that the maintenance of a healthy body and mind is important, both in reducing the chances of developing an infection and in speeding recovery. It also seems logical that medicines that interfere with the natural defences of the body (e.g. antipyretic, anti-emetic and anti-inflammatory drugs) should be used with caution. Have you noticed how many Western medicines start with 'anti'?

Recurrent infections

Sometimes patients present with a history of several different types of infection over a short period of time.

In such cases, consider:
- increased exposure to infections (e.g. child starting school)
- psychosocial stress (a potent immunosuppressant)
- white cell dysfunction (e.g. leukaemia – full blood count)
- diabetes (fasting blood glucose)
- HIV (serology, with counselling and leaflet beforehand)
- immunoglobulins, in children and young people

TABLE 11.1 Some of the bacteria which cause common infections, and the antibiotics most frequently used against them

Organism	Commensal	Diseases	Antibiotic susceptibility
Streptococcus	Throat	Pharyngitis, otitis media, pneumonia, meningitis, cellulitis, impetigo	**Phenoxymethylpenicillin,** amoxicillin, clarithromycin
Staphylococcus	Nose	Impetigo, boils, abscesses, cellulitis	**Flucloxacillin,** clarithromycin
Haemophilus influenzae	Upper respiratory tract	Otitis media, epiglottitis, meningitis, chest infections	**Amoxicillin** (80%), co-amoxiclav, clarithromycin, doxycycline
Escherichia coli	Intestine	UTI, abscesses, gastro-enteritis	**Trimethoprim** (70%), nitrofurantoin, cefalexin

References

Guarner F, Malgelada JR. Gut flora in health and disease. *Lancet.* 2003; **361**: 512–19.

Pedersen E, Zachariae R, Bovbjerg D. Influence of psychosocial stress on upper respiratory infections – a meta-analysis of prospective studies. *Psychosom Med.* 2010; **72**: 823–32.

Notifiable diseases

Diseases which must be notified to the local Health Protection Unit (HPU) on the appropriate form include:

- suspected food poisoning
- measles
- mumps
- rubella
- pertussis
- scarlet fever
- chickenpox (in Scotland)

A full list is given on the cover of the book of notification forms. This notification is statutory and does not require the patient's consent. Warn the patient that he or she may be contacted by the local HPU, and explain that their role is to identify the source of infections and prevent their spread. If there are any implications for the community, e.g. suspected food poisoning in a chef or a rare infectious disease, notify the local consultant in communicable disease by telephone.

References

Health Protection Agency. *Patient Confidentiality – Caldicott.* London: Health Protection Agency; 2005. Available at: www.hpa.org.uk

Health Protection Agency. *Guidance on Infection Control in Schools and Other Childcare Settings.* London: Health Protection Agency; 2010. Available at: www.hpa.org.uk

Health Protection Agency. *Guidance on Viral Rash in Pregnancy: investigation, diagnosis and management of viral rash illness, or exposure to viral rash illness in pregnancy.* London: Health Protection Agency; 2011. Available at: www.hpa.org.uk

TABLE 11.2 Infectiousness and exclusion periods for common diseases

Disease/infection	Incubation period	Infective period	Exclusion from school	Action for contacts
Chickenpox	11–20 days	From 1 day before until 5 days from onset of rash	5 days after rash appears	Refer babies under 4 weeks, non-immune immunosuppressed or pregnant contacts
Conjunctivitis	3–29 days	While discharge present	None	None
Cryptosporidium	2–5 days	While diarrhoea lasts	Until 48 h after last diarrhoea or vomiting. No swimming for 2 weeks	HPU will decide
Diarrhoea and vomiting	1 hour–14 days (depending on cause)	While diarrhoea lasts	Until 48 h after last diarrhoea or vomiting	No exclusion unless bacterial cause, when HPU will decide
Glandular fever	33–49 days	None	Until well	None
Hand, foot and mouth disease	3–5 days	Up to 7 days	None	None
Head lice	7–10 days	As long as lice or live eggs are present	Until treated	None
Impetigo	Unknown	While purulent lesions persist	Until lesions crusted, or 48 h after treatment begun	None
Measles	6–19 days	From 4 days before onset of rash to 4 days after	4 days	Refer non-immune immunosuppressed or pregnant contacts
Mumps	15–24 days	From 6 days before symptoms to 4 days after onset	5 days	None
Parvovirus (slapped cheek)	13–18 days	Until rash appears	None	Refer pregnant contacts under 30 weeks
Pertussis (whooping cough)	5–21 days	Up to 3 weeks if untreated	5 days after starting antibiotic, or 3 weeks if no antibiotic	Consult HPU
Rubella	13–21 days	From 13 days before rash until 6 days after	6 days	Refer non-immune pregnant contacts under 20 weeks
Scabies	7–27 days	Until mites and eggs have been destroyed	After treatment	None once treated

(continued)

Disease/infection	Incubation period	Infective period	Exclusion from school	Action for contacts
Scarlet fever	12 h to 5 days	Up to 24 h after antibiotic	24 h after first antibiotic treatment	None
Shingles	None	Until 5 days after onset of rash	None, provided lesions covered	Refer babies under 4 weeks, non-immune immunosuppressed or pregnant contacts if exposed to uncovered lesions
Threadworms	2–6 weeks	As long as eggs present	None once treated	None once treated
Tinea	1–2 weeks	While lesions are active	None	None
Verrucas (plantar warts)	1–24 months	as long as wart present	None (cover wart with waterproof dressing for swimming/barefoot sports)	None

Source: Health Protection Agency, 2010

Certificates

NHS certificates (fit notes)

- are not issued for periods of less than 7 calendar days; these patients should obtain a Self Certification (SC2) form from their employer, or an SC1 form if self-employed or unemployed. See www.direct.gov.uk.
- do not require face-to-face assessment
- may be completed after telephone consultation
- may be based on a written report by another registered healthcare professional (e.g. computer entry by minor illness nurse, or fax from an urgent care centre)
- may be used to state that the patient is unfit for any work
- alternatively, the patient may be certified fit for limited work:
  — phased return
  — altered hours
  — amended duties
  — workplace adaptations
  — other (in 'comments' box), e.g. time off to attend appointments
- choice of 'open' statements (this will be the case for . . .) and 'closed' statements (from . . . to . . .)
- use closed statements:
  — if the period is less than 14 days, and
  — the patient does not need to be reassessed
- cannot be forward-dated, although overlapping is permitted
- closed statements can be backdated

Reference

Department for Work and Pensions. *Sick Note to Fit note.* www.dwp.gov.uk/fitnote

Private certificates

These can be issued by GP practices at their discretion. There will be a fee, which should be reclaimed from the employer.

12

Minor illness formulary

This formulary aims to cover the range of medication commonly required to treat minor illness. You may wish to adapt it in light of your local formulary, prescribing policy or Patient Group Directions.

The formulary gives information on the clinical use of medications and the justification for recommending such medication. The *British National Formulary* (*BNF*), *British National Formulary for Children* (*BNFC*) and their appendices, or the Summary of Product Characteristics (SPC) provide more information online (http://bnf.org or http://bnfc.org and www.medicines.org.uk). As a final check before giving a prescription, the acronym *PASS* can be used to check if the patient is *Pregnant*, *Allergic*, on *Something else*, or has a *System failure*. When considering if a patient is pregnant, bear in mind that those hoping to become pregnant but who have not yet missed a period and mothers who are breastfeeding also need special caution when prescribing. Always check for interaction with any other current medication. Some drugs are contraindicated (i.e. should not be used) in, or should be given at lower dosage to, patients with kidney, liver or heart failure. Information on this is given in the section notes of the *BNF* and in the individual drug entries. If in doubt, ask an experienced doctor.

Notes on prescribing

Above all, make sure the prescription specifies the drug you intended. Most prescriptions in primary care are now computer-printed. The difference between drugs with similarly spelt names can be as little as the gap between two adjacent keys on a keyboard. One of the most dangerous examples is prescribing penicillamine when penicillin was intended. Such an inadvertent swap from an antibiotic to an immunosuppressant could be fatal.

If you do need to write a prescription by hand, be aware of some additional pitfalls. The prescription form has a box at the top where the number of days' treatment may be entered. This avoids the need to calculate quantities but is awkward to use. It cannot be used for variable-dose drugs, creams, lotions, etc. Remember that the box is an instruction to the pharmacist as to how much to dispense, not a direction to the patient, so it will not appear on the dispensed medication instructions unless repeated in the main body of the prescription. On the whole, it is usually simpler and clearer to specify an amount to be dispensed and leave the top box blank.

Clear, uncluttered prescriptions are safest. Try to avoid decimal points (e.g. 500 mg is preferable to 0.5 g), repeating words, using superfluous words, or adding instructions that will be on the medication label anyway. To discover the cautionary and advisory label, look up the drug in the *BNF* and find the label number near the end of the entry, then check the corresponding text on the last page inside the back cover. Further information is given in Appendix 3 of the *BNF*.

Previous antibiotic treatment

If a patient presents with a condition requiring antibiotic treatment, but has finished a course of the 'first-choice' antibiotic within the last 7 days, then either the infection is viral or the organism is resistant to the antibiotic. In these circumstances, a different antibiotic may be necessary, as follows:

- for otitis media or sinusitis – change to co-amoxiclav
- for chest infections – add clarithromycin or change to doxycycline
- for uncomplicated urinary tract infections in non-pregnant women – change to either nitrofurantoin m/r or trimethoprim, whichever one was not used last time (unless sensitivities are available from the laboratory)
- for throat infections – take throat swab and await result before prescribing a different antibiotic, as in most cases the infection will be viral

Antibiotics and oral contraceptives

None of the antibiotics in this formulary interact with oral contraceptives. In fact the only antibiotics that do interact are the few that enhance the action of enzymes, such as some used to treat tuberculosis. There is no need to advise women to change their normal pill routine.

References

British National Formulary. *7.3.1 Combined Hormonal Contraceptives*. Available at: http://bnf. org/bnf/bnf/current/4552.htm (accessed 28 November 2011).

Faculty of Sexual and Reproductive Healthcare Clinical Effectiveness Unit. *Drug Interactions with Hormonal Contraception*. 2011. Available at: www.fsrh.org/pdfs/CEUGuidanceDrug InteractionsHormonal.pdf (accessed 15 November 2011).

Absorption

Not surprisingly, tablets and capsules are designed to dissolve, and dissolve very fast in the hot acid environment of the stomach. There is no need to prescribe liquid or dispersible medication in an attempt to speed up absorption. Solids are preferable, being chemically more stable and less expensive. Even in acute migraine, when the stomach may be immobile, the average difference in speed of absorption between tablets and liquid is only 10 minutes. Some tablets dissolve on the tongue, but the resulting liquid still needs to be swallowed. This is not for speed of onset, but when ordinary tablets cannot be swallowed easily, for example, when there is no ready access to water.

Modified-release tablets are designed to dissolve slowly to give a prolonged effect or reduced side-effects. Enteric coating is a way of protecting a drug from damage by gastric acid. The coating resists acid but dissolves in the more alkaline small bowel, the site of absorption of almost all oral drugs. Note that enteric coating protects the drug, not the patient's stomach. Gastric side-effects are usually due to the overall effect of a drug after it has been absorbed, so the route by which it is given is immaterial. A non-steroidal anti-inflammatory drug can cause a gastric bleed from the action of the drug, whether it is given orally, rectally or by injection.

Half-life ($t_{1/2}$)

The speed at which a drug is eliminated from the body is often proportional to the concentration of drug in the blood. When the drug is present in high concentration shortly after a dose, the elimination is more rapid than when it is present only in low concentration some time later. Drugs that follow this rule are said to have first-order kinetics, and they have a constant half-life. When this is so, the plasma half-life is given in this formulary. This is the time taken for the plasma concentration of the drug to reduce by one half of its starting level. It is useful to know the $t_{1/2}$, even if it is only an approximation, to help understand how long the action of a drug will last and when a further dose may be needed. When there is a known range of $t_{1/2}$ for different individuals, this is given in brackets after the mean.

Allergies

Many reported allergies are really just coincidences, for example, the appearance of a viral rash just after starting a course of antibiotic. However, any report of swelling of the tongue or face, or difficulty in breathing, must be taken seriously.

Allergic reactions are usually:

- itchy
- generalised
- confluent
- within 3 days of taking the drug, sometimes later

If the patient has a true allergy to one type of penicillin, *all* drugs of this class should be avoided. This does not apply if the patient experiences non-allergic side-effects, such as diarrhoea with co-amoxiclav; penicillin V will probably not produce this side-effect.

True penicillin allergy occurs in 7%–23% of people who say they are allergic to penicillin. The frequently cited figure of 10% cross-reactivity between penicillin and cephalosporins is an overestimate (early cephalosporins were contaminated with penicillin moulds). The true figure is more like 0.5%. There may be a higher rate of cross-reactivity with completely unrelated antibiotics.

Reference

Pegler S, Healy B. In patients allergic to penicillin, consider second and third generation cephalosporins for life threatening infections. *BMJ*. 2007; **335**: 991.

Adverse drug reactions

Adverse drug reactions (ADR), often referred to as 'side-effects', are very common and becoming more so with increasing prescribing to prevent or control long-term conditions. They account for 6.5% of acute admissions to hospital, rising to around 10% of admissions to wards for medical care of older patients. We found no recent research into the impact of such reactions on primary care consultations, but our experience at the National Minor Illness Centre is that in about one in 30 consultations, the presenting symptom is a result of an unwanted effect of medication. This equates to about one a day for a specialist clinician in minor illness. Thus it is essential to consider acute symptoms in light of concurrent medication. If an ADR is suspected, the principle to follow is that it is far better to stop or change a medication that is causing problems than start another to control the unwanted effects. However, this is not always possible. If you do not normally prescribe the medication in question, seek advice from a clinician who does.

Interactions

A simple theoretical model, based purely on probability, shows that if the chance of an interaction between any two drugs is 1%, the chance of an interaction occurring when someone is taking 12 drugs is about 50%. Thus without careful selection, prescribing for an acute condition in such a patient would stand a 1-in-2 chance of interacting with a pre-existing medication. Fortunately, many interactions are not serious; the prime aim is to avoid those that are. Warnings from clinical computer systems are helpful, but if you find your attention to such alerts wanes because of their frequency, consider changing the user settings to only alert you to a higher-priority problem.

Be particularly cautious when the long-term medication includes:
- aspirin
- amiodarone
- antiepileptics
- antipsychotics
- ciclosporin
- digoxin
- lithium
- methotrexate
- monoamine-oxidase inhibitor antidepressants
- St John's wort
- theophylline
- warfarin

OTC

Drugs marked 'OTC' are available over the counter, and often cost less than a prescription charge. The price depends on the pack size, brand and pharmacy.

▼Black triangle symbol

This symbol means that there is limited experience of the use of this product and the Medicines and Healthcare Products Regulatory Agency (MRHA) requests that *all* suspected adverse reactions should be reported. Use the yellow forms in the *BNF*. They can be signed and submitted by any health professional, not just doctors. An online version can be found at http://yellowcard.mhra.gov.uk.

◣ Less suitable for prescribing symbol

This symbol means that the Joint Formulary Committee of the *BNF* considers a drug to be 'less suitable for prescribing'. Several are in fairly common use in managing minor illnesses despite this. If you feel tempted to use a drug not in our formulary, it is worth checking to see if the *BNF* lists the drug with this symbol. If it does, then there is usually either an unacceptable balance between efficacy and side-effects, or the drug is simply considered ineffective.

Formulations

Only the formulations of the drugs suitable for the indications described in the main text of this book are listed. Others may be available, but for other indications.

Pack size

The number of tablets, capsules or items, or the volume of liquids is given in the formulary for the usual original pack dispensed. This is not to be taken as a recommendation of how much to prescribe, which depends on the patient's needs, but when possible it is more convenient for a manufactured pack to be dispensed whole, together with the patient information leaflet.

Dosage

Only the doses relevant to prescribing for minor illness are listed in the formulary. Other dosages and formulations may be available.

Prescribing for children

Children are not just small adults; like everything else, their chemistry is still developing and they may handle drugs quite differently. Some drugs that are safe for use by adults cannot be taken by children because of the risk of a side-effect that only affects children – for example, aspirin may cause Reye's syndrome. For drugs that can be prescribed for children, the dose is usually calculated by weight. This may not be the best method, but it is practical.

Tips for safe prescribing for children:
- use the *BNFC*
- calculate the dose from the child's weight
- have an approximate idea of what the likely dose is to check the calculation is correct, or compare it with a dose for a given age range
- note the instruction on how many doses per day

If no weighing scales are available, use the age-range dose in the *BNFC* or calculate according to the average weight-for-age table near the back of the book. As a last resort, an approximate weight can be calculated as (age + 4) × 2 kg, so a 6-year-old would weigh about 20 kg. This will give a weight to within 15% of the normal weight of a child of that age.

If you suspect an adverse drug reaction in anyone under the age of 18 years, it should be reported to the *MRHA* using the yellow form in the back of the *BNF* or online (see above). This is because experience of use of the drug in children may still be limited.

Prescribing in pregnancy and breastfeeding

Every prescriber tries to avoid prescribing in pregnancy, but sometimes the risk from medication is outweighed by a greater risk of leaving a condition untreated, such as a urinary infection. Nurse Independent Prescribers are able to prescribe any medicine for any medical condition, including those presenting in pregnancy, so long as they work within their own level of professional competence and expertise. Before prescribing, always check the entry of the drug in the *BNF* that identifies drugs which may have harmful effects in pregnancy and indicates the trimester of risk. Similar caution is needed in breastfeeding.

Routes of drug administration

Take advantage of the wide range of formulations of drugs. If a patient would benefit from a particular medication but there is potential risk or difficulty, consider using the drug via a different route of administration to the usual one, rather than changing to a less appropriate treatment. For example, a patient with a history of a peptic ulcer could use a topical NSAID for a soft-tissue injury, whereas oral treatment would be unwise. Be aware that occasionally an unusual formulation may be much more expensive than the usual one. At the time of publication, the drug tariff price of a standard pack of nitrofurantoin m/r is £4.89 compared with a bottle of nitrofurantoin liquid at £99, and paracetamol tablets are a penny each compared with £1 for a paracetamol suppository. Check the price of generic drugs online at www.ppa.org.uk/ppa/edt_intro.htm in Part VIII, 'Basic Prices of Drugs Product List'. The latest edition of *MIMS* will give an up-to-date price of branded products, but the *BNF* price may be somewhat out-of-date. If you cannot find a particular form of a medicine in the *BNF* at all, it may be available but only supplied as a 'special' drug, without a set price, that could turn out to be thousands of pounds.

Formulary

Formulary listed by *BNF* classification.

Gastrointestinal system

Mucogel [1.1]
Gaviscon Advance [1.1.2]
Ranitidine [1.3.1]
Omeprazole [1.3.5]
Loperamide [1.4.2]
Fybogel [1.6.1]
Glycerol suppositories [1.6.2]
Senna [1.6.2]
Movicol [1.6.4]
Anusol [1.7.1]
Xyloproct [1.7.2]

Cardiovascular system

Nifedipine [2.6.2]
Tranexamic acid [2.11]

Respiratory system

Salbutamol [3.1.1]
Spacer devices [3.1.5]
Peak flow meter [3.1.5]
Beclometasone [3.2]
Cetirizine [3.4.1]
Loratadine [3.4.1]
Chlorphenamine [3.4.1]
Menthol and eucalyptus [3.8]
Simple linctus [3.9.2]

Nervous system

Temazepam [4.1.1]
Prochlorperazine [4.6]
Domperidone [4.6]
Aspirin [4.7.1]
Paracetamol [4.7.1]
Codeine phosphate [4.7.2]
Sumatriptan [4.7.4]

Infection

Phenoxymethylpenicillin [5.1.1]
Flucloxacillin [5.1.1.2]
Amoxicillin [5.1.1.3]
Co-amoxiclav [5.1.1.3]
Cefalexin [5.1.2]
Doxycycline [5.1.3]
Erythromycin [5.1.5]
Azithromycin [5.1.5]
Clarithromycin [5.1.5]
Trimethoprim [5.1.8]
Metronidazole [5.1.11]
Nitrofurantoin m/r [5.1.13]
Fluconazole [5.2.1]
Aciclovir [5.3.2.1]
Mebendazole [5.5.1]
Piperazine + senna [5.5.1]

Endocrine system

Prednisolone [6.3.2]
Norethisterone [6.4.1.2]

Obstetrics and gynaecology

Clotrimazole [7.2.2]
Metronidazole [7.2.2]
Clindamycin [7.2.2]
Levonorgestrel [7.3.5]
Ulipristal [7.3.5]

Nutrition and blood

Ferrous sulphate [9.1.1]
Dioralyte [9.2.1.2]

Musculoskeletal system

Ibuprofen [10.1.1]
Naproxen [10.1.1]
Ketoprofen topical [10.3.2]

Eye

Chloramphenicol [11.3.1]
Fusidic acid [11.3.1]
Azelastine [11.4.2]
Sodium cromoglicate [11.4.2]
Viscotears [11.8.1]

Ear, nose and oropharynx

EarCalm [12.1.1]
Otosporin [12.1.1]
Locorten-Vioform [12.1.1]
Otomize [12.1.1]
Azelastine [12.2.1]
Rhinocort Aqua [12.2.1]
Sodium chloride: Stérimar [12.2.2]
Water vapour inhalation [12.2.2]
Ephedrine nose drops [12.2.2]
Benzydamine [12.3.1]
Hydrocortisone [12.3.1]
Miconazole [12.3.2]
Chlorhexidine [12.3.4]

Skin

Aqueous cream [13.2.1]
Emulsifying ointment [13.2.1]
Hydrous ointment [13.2.1]
Paraffin, yellow soft BP [13.2.1]
Cetraben [13.2.1]
E45 lotion [13.2.1]
QV bath oil [13.2.1.1]
Hydromol [13.2.1.1]
Metanium [13.2.2]
Crotamiton [13.3]
Hydrocortisone [13.4]
Eumovate [13.4]
Betnovate RD [13.4]
Betnovate [13.4]
Canesten HC [13.4]
Benzoyl peroxide [13.6.1]
Duac [13.6.1]
Azelaic acid [13.6.1]
Zineryt [13.6.1]

Tretinoin [13.6.1]
Salactol [13.7]
Ketoconazole [13.9]
Capasal [13.9]
Sodium fusidate [13.10.1]
Clotrimazole [13.10.2]
Terbinafine [13.10.2]
Aciclovir [13.10.3]
Dimeticone [13.10.4]
Malathion [13.10.4]
Permethrin [13.10.4]

Borderline substances

SMA LF [A2.3.1]

Gastrointestinal system

[1.1] Mucogel® (OTC)

Class:	antacid
Suspension:	sugar-free co-magaldrox
Dose:	adults and children over 12 years: 10–20 mL 3 times daily, 20–60 minutes after meals and at bedtime or when required
Pack:	500 mL
Side-effects:	the balance of magnesium and aluminium hydroxides minimises the problems of diarrhoea and constipation
Interactions:	may reduce the absorption of other drugs; for example, tetracyclines, ciprofloxacin, lansoprazole, vitamins, fexofenadine, digoxin, phenytoin
Cautions:	avoid in renal failure
Selection:	antacids provide rapid, short-term relief from dyspepsia. Plain alkali can cause rebound acid secretion, but magnesium and aluminium salts are insoluble in water and may be retained in the stomach longer to protect the gastric mucosa. Liquid preparations are more effective than tablets

[1.1.2] Gaviscon Advance® (OTC)

Class:	compound alginate antacid
Liquid:	sodium alginate 500 mg, potassium bicarbonate 100 mg per 5 mL
Dose:	adults and children over 12 years: 5–10 mL after meals and at bedtime
Pack:	250, 500 mL
Side-effects:	very rarely, patients sensitive to the ingredients may develop allergic manifestations such as urticaria or bronchospasm
Interactions:	as the protective gel is formed by the alginate and bicarbonate reacting with gastric acid to produce a froth of mucoid carbon dioxide bubbles, other medication that reduces gastric acid secretion may make a less effective raft, but clinical trials have found little effect on efficacy
Cautions:	the salts of sodium, potassium and calcium (an excipient in Gaviscon Advance) might exacerbate some severe diseases, such as cardiac failure, hyperkalaemia, calcium-containing renal stones
Selection:	whereas co-magaldrox primarily reduces acidity and forms a barrier to protect the gastric mucosa, compound alginate agents such as Gaviscon Advance form a raft to reduce the chance that acid can reflux up into the oesophagus, which helps to control the symptoms of mild to moderate heartburn. The Advance version has a lower sodium content than plain Gaviscon (still available for infants), and is no more expensive. It can be used in pregnancy

References

Chatfield S. A comparison of the efficacy of the alginate preparation, Gaviscon Advance, with placebo in the treatment of gastro-oesophageal reflux disease. *Curr Med Res Opin*. 1999; **15**: 152–9.

Lindow SW, Regnèll P, Sykes J, *et al*. An open-label, multicentre study to assess the safety and efficacy of a novel reflux suppressant Gaviscon Advance in the treatment of heartburn during pregnancy. *Int J Clin Pract*. 2003; **57**: 175–9.

[1.3.1] Ranitidine (lower-dose tablets available OTC)

for use in allergy where conventional antihistamines are insufficient

Class:	histamine H_2 receptor blocker
Tablets:	150, 300 mg
Dose:	150 mg twice daily or 300 mg at night
Pack:	60 × 150 mg; 30 × 300 mg
$t_{1/2}$:	2 h
Side-effects:	ranitidine is usually well tolerated, but very rarely is associated with changes in liver or kidney function, pancreatitis, reduction in white cell or platelet counts, bradycardia, headache, allergic phenomena such as rash, joint aches or vasculitis
Interactions:	the reduction in gastric acidity can affect the absorption of other drugs, but this is clinically significant only for drugs where the absorption is markedly acid-dependent or the dose absorbed is critical: warfarin, ulipristal, midazolam, glipizide and the oral antifungals itraconazole, ketoconazole and posaconazole
Cautions:	use half the normal dose in severe renal impairment (eGFR < 50 mL/min). Do not prescribe for people with a history of acute porphyria
Selection:	when blocking H_1 receptors by conventional antihistamines such as cetirizine or loratadine has failed to relieve allergic symptoms adequately, one option is to *add in* ranitidine to block H_2 receptors as well in case the patient has an unusually high proportion of these involved in their allergic response. Warn the patient that the information leaflet they will find in the pack will describe effects on the stomach, but that is not why they are taking the medication. Ranitidine rarely causes side-effects. Effervescent or liquid preparations are much more expensive. Cimetidine is also more expensive, has undesirable anti-androgenic effects and multiple drug interactions

References

Grattan C, Powell S, Humphreys F. Management and diagnostic guidelines for urticaria and angio-oedema. *Br J Dermatol*. 2001; **144**: 708–14.

Lin RY, Curry A, Pesola GR, *et al.* Improved outcomes in patients with acute allergic syndromes who are treated with combined H_1 and H_2 antagonists. *Ann Emerg Med*. 2000; **36**(5): 462–8.

[1.3.5] Omeprazole (10 mg tablets available OTC)

Class:	proton pump inhibitor
Enteric-coated capsules:	10, 20 mg
Dose:	adults: 20 mg once daily to protect against peptic ulcer while taking NSAID; for dyspepsia 20 mg once daily and review after 4 weeks
Pack:	28
$t_{1/2}$:	less than 1 h, but the inhibition of gastric acidity (pH $\geq$ 3) lasts a mean of 17 h
Side-effects:	proton pump inhibitors are potent inhibitors of gastric acid secretion. Although they are usually well tolerated, there are risks associated with the use of these drugs that do not give rise to symptoms but increase the risk of developing significant diseases, such as gastrointestinal infections including *Clostridium difficile*, osteoporosis and pneumonia. Gastrointestinal side-effects (abdominal pain, constipation, diarrhoea, flatulence, nausea, vomiting) are relatively common, as is headache. Less frequently, dry mouth, oedema, dizziness, tiredness and sleep disturbances, paraesthesia, arthralgia, myalgia, rash and pruritus. Rarely, taste disturbance, stomatitis, hepatitis, allergic reactions, fever, depression, hallucinations, confusion, gynaecomastia, interstitial nephritis, hyponatraemia, blood disorders, visual disturbances, sweating, photosensitivity, alopecia
Interactions:	**antacids** should not be taken within 2 h of a dose as they may affect the enteric coating of the capsule; ciclosporin, clarithromycin, **clopidogrel**, diazepam, digoxin, escitalopram, itraconazole, ketoconazole, methotrexate, phenytoin, posaconazole, St John's wort, tacrolimus, **ulipristal**, warfarin
Cautions:	do not assume that resolution of symptoms in response to omeprazole can be diagnostically reassuring. Proton pump inhibitors can mask the symptoms of gastric cancer
Selection:	omeprazole is the most cost-effective proton pump inhibitor. Prescribe the capsules, as the tablets are more expensive for no benefit. Omeprazole is not known to be harmful in pregnancy or breastfeeding. Use a proton pump inhibitor only when necessary, as there are associated risks that will not be recognized by the patient and there can be acid-related symptoms on withdrawal of therapy even in people who had no symptoms prior to treatment

References

Forgacs I, Loganayagam A. Overprescribing proton pump inhibitors. *BMJ*. 2008; **336**: 2–3.

Heidelbaugh JJ, Goldberg KL, Inadomi JM. Adverse risks associated with proton pump inhibitors: a systematic review. *Gastroenterol Hepatol (N Y)*. 2009; **5**: 725–34.

Reimer C, Søndergaard B, Hilsted L, *et al*. Proton-pump inhibitor therapy induces acid-related symptoms in healthy volunteers after withdrawal of therapy. *Gastroenterology*. 2009; **137**: 80–7, 87.e1.

[1.4.2] Loperamide (OTC)

Class:	antimotility opioid
Capsules:	2 mg
Dose:	adults: 2 capsules initially, followed by 1 after each loose stool for up to a maximum of 5 days; usual dose 3–4 capsules a day, maximum of 8 capsules a day
Pack:	30
$t_{1/2}$:	11 (9–14) h
Side-effects:	abdominal cramps, bloating, nausea, vomiting and rarely paralytic ileus, dizziness, drowsiness, skin reactions
Interactions:	oral desmopressin
Cautions:	avoid in abdominal distension, active ulcerative colitis, bloody diarrhoea, pregnancy; not suitable for children (although licensed from age 4), or anyone with undiagnosed abdominal pain, risk of accumulation in severe liver disease
Selection:	loperamide provides rapid relief from diarrhoea – within 4 h for 40% of people with traveller's diarrhoea

References

Steffen R, Heusser R, Tschopp A, *et al*. Efficacy and side-effects of six agents in the self-treatment of traveller's diarrhoea. *Travel Med Int*. 1988; **6**: 153–7.

Wingate D, Phillips SF, Lewis SJ, *et al*. Guidelines for adults on self-medication for the treatment of acute diarrhoea. *Aliment Pharmacol Ther*. 2001; **15**: 773–82.

[1.6.1] Fybogel® (OTC)

Class:	bulk-forming laxative
Granules:	effervescent sugar- and gluten-free ispaghul husk, 3.5 g/sachet, (plain, lemon or orange flavour)
Dose:	adults: 1 sachet in water twice daily, preferably after or with meals child 6–12 years: ½ sachet twice daily, preferably after or with meals
Pack:	30
Side-effects:	flatulence, abdominal distension, gastrointestinal obstruction or impaction, very rarely allergic reactions
Interactions:	none
Cautions:	adequate liquid intake is essential to reduce the risk of intestinal obstruction. In vitro, the husk can absorb up to 40 times its own weight of water. Do not prescribe for patients with difficulty swallowing, intestinal obstruction or atony, or faecal impaction
Selection:	the best form of medicine for constipation is to increase the natural fibre in the diet. When this is not achievable, bulk-forming laxatives are an alternative. Ispaghul husk is also useful for controlling diarrhoea in diverticular disease and when there is too much fluid in an ileostomy or colostomy. At first, this seems paradoxical, but it is just making use of the liquid-absorbing property of the husk

Reference

Dettmar PW, Sykes J. A multi-centre, general practice comparison of ispaghula husk with lactulose and other laxatives in the treatment of simple constipation. *Curr Med Res Opin*. 1998; **14**: 227–33.

[1.6.2] Glycerol suppositories (OTC)

Class: lubricant and mildly stimulant rectal laxative

Suppositories: gelatine 140 mg/g, glycerol 700 mg/g, purified water 160 mg/g

Dose: adults and children over 12 years: 4 g

children 1–12 years: 2 g

1 month–1 year: 1 g

insert one suppository, blunt end first, into the rectum when required

Pack: 12

Side-effects: rectal discomfort

Interactions: none

Selection: glycerol is a simple, safe laxative suitable for short-term relief of distal constipation

Reference

Abd-El-Maeboud KH, El-Naggar T, El-Hawi EM, *et al*. Rectal suppository: commonsense and mode of insertion. *Lancet*. 1991; **338**(8770): 798–800.

[1.6.2] Senna (OTC)

Class:	stimulant laxative
Tablets:	7.5 mg (for adults and children over 6 years)
Syrup:	7.5 mg/5 mL
Dose:	start with the lowest dose in the range, then increase if necessary:
	adults and children over 18 years: 15–30 mg at night
	children 6–18 years: 7.5–30 mg at night *or* in the morning
	4–6 years: 3.75–30 mg in the morning
	2–4 years: 3.75–15 mg in the morning
Pack:	60 tablets; 100 mL
Side-effects:	abdominal cramp, prolonged use can cause an atonic, non-functioning colon and hypokalaemia
Interactions:	none
Cautions:	do not prescribe to patients with intestinal obstruction. Long-term use has risks but is sometimes justified. Young children with chronic constipation should be referred to a doctor
Selection:	stimulant laxatives may be necessary to relieve generalised constipation where diet or a bulk-forming laxative has failed and glycerol would not help evacuate the colon. The action of senna takes about 8–12 h. It is best administered after the stool has been softened by other measures: increased dietary fibre and water intake, or an osmotic laxative such as Movicol. Fears over a link between senna use and colonic cancer are unsupported by evidence

Reference

Leung L, Riutta T, Kotecha J, *et al.* Chronic constipation: an evidence-based review. *J Am Board Fam Med.* 2011; **24**: 436–51.

[1.6.4] Movicol® (OTC) and Movicol® Paediatric Plain

Class:	osmotic laxative
Oral powder sachets:	macrogol '3350', sodium bicarbonate, sodium chloride, potassium chloride
Dose:	for chronic constipation:
	adults and children over 12: 1 sachet 1–3 times daily, reducing the dose according to the response within 2 weeks to the usual maintain dose of 1 sachet once or twice daily
	Paediatric Plain: children 6–12 years, 2 Paediatric Plain sachets daily, adjusted according to response (max. 4 sachets daily); 1–6 years, 1 Paediatric Plain sachet daily, adjusted according to response (max. 4 sachets daily); under 1 year, ½–1 Paediatric Plain sachet daily
Pack:	30
Side-effects:	diarrhoea, abdominal distension, vomiting, nausea, anal discomfort – all tend to be with the higher dose range
Interactions:	there is a possibility that tablets or capsules, especially enteric-coated or modified-release preparations, taken within 1 h of Movicol could be flushed through the gut, reducing absorption
Cautions:	do not prescribe for patients with difficulty swallowing, intestinal obstruction or atony, or active inflammatory bowel disease. Avoid in cardiovascular or renal disease as there is no information available
Selection:	Movicol Paediatric Plain is the only macrogol licensed for children under 12 years that includes electrolytes and not flavouring

References

Candy DC, Edwards D, Geraint M. Treatment of faecal impaction with polyethelene glycol plus electrolytes (PGE + E) followed by a double-blind comparison of PEG + E versus lactulose as maintenance therapy. *J Pediatr Gastroenterol Nutr*. 2006; **43**: 65–70.

Dupont C, Leluyer B, Maamri N, *et al*. Double-blind randomized evaluation of clinical and biological tolerance of polyethylene glycol 4000 versus lactulose in constipated children. *J Pediatr Gastroenterol Nutr*. 2005; **41**: 625–33.

[1.7.1] Anusol® (OTC)

Class:	soothing haemorrhoidal preparation
Ointment:	bismuth subgallate 2.25%, bismuth oxide 0.88%, balsam peru 1.88%, zinc oxide 10.75% Suppositories: similar proportions of above in a 2.8 g suppository
Dose:	1 suppository or application of ointment night and morning and after defecation
Pack:	12, 24 suppositories, 25 g of ointment
Side-effects:	rarely discomfort on application or local dermatitis
Interactions:	none
Cautions:	avoid prescribing to patients who are sensitive to lanolin as this is one of the excipients
Selection:	Anusol exerts its effects locally without systemic absorption. Although no formal trials in pregnancy have been done, it has been used during pregnancy for many years and is considered safe. The ointment is used for external haemorrhoids and may provide better protection and lubrication of the anal surface than a cream. Suppositories are used for internal haemorrhoids

[1.7.2] Xyloproct®

Class:	soothing haemorrhoidal preparation with corticosteroid and local anaesthetic
Ointment:	aluminium acetate 3.5%, hydrocortisone acetate 0.275%, lidocaine 5%, zinc oxide 18%
Dose:	apply several times daily
Pack:	20 g (with applicator)
Side-effects:	stinging on application, local dermatitis, very rarely systemic effects from absorption of the components, with confusions in children or hypersensitivity reactions
Cautions:	pregnancy, anal infections such as herpes simplex or candida. Avoid prolonged use which could theoretically result in local skin atrophy from the hydrocortisone. It would be very unusual to prescribe this for a child
Selection:	the idea is that the corticosteroid controls itching and the lidocaine controls the pain. The aluminium acetate is a soothing component. An applicator is supplied so that the ointment can be applied within the rectum if required. The usual indication is painful or irritant haemorrhoids, but the preparation is also useful for symptomatic relief from an anal fissure or troublesome pruritus ani

Cardiovascular system

[2.6.2] Nifedipine

Class:	calcium channel blocker
Capsules:	5 mg
Dose:	lactating women with Raynaud's disease of nipple: 5 mg 3 times daily for 2 weeks
Pack:	84
$t_{1/2}$:	1.7 to 3.4 h
Side-effects:	at this very low dose taken for just 2 weeks, side-effects are unlikely, but could include disturbance of gut function, lightheadedness, oedema, flushing, palpitations, headache, lethargy; occasionally nasal congestion, dyspnoea, anxiety, sleep disturbance, vertigo, migraine, paraesthesia, tremor, polyuria, dysuria, nocturia, epistaxis, myalgia, joint swelling, visual disturbance, sweating, allergic reactions, impaired glucose tolerance
Interactions:	enhanced hypotension if taken with other drugs that lower blood pressure: antihypertensives especially beta-blockers, alcohol, antipsychotics, anxiolytics and hypnotics, baclofen, clonidine, levodopa, MAOI antidepressants, nitrates, vardenafil; theophylline, digoxin, tacrolimus or dronedarone levels may be increased; fluoxetine, grapefruit juice may increase effect of nifedipine
Cautions:	cardiovascular disease is unlikely given the indication for nifedipine in this formulary, but if present it would be essential to seek advice from an experienced prescriber; avoid in pregnancy; monitor glucose in diabetes; may be used with caution in porphyria
Selection:	nifedipine is a first-line treatment for Raynaud's phenomenon as it improves peripheral circulation by vasodilation. Here it is suggested for the specific indication of Raynaud's disease of the nipple in lactation. The manufacturer advises against using the drug in breastfeeding, but the amount secreted into the milk is too low to be harmful. Advise the woman to avoid starting to breastfeed when the nipple is cold, and, if smoking, ideally quit as the nicotine will exacerbate the problem

Reference

Anderson JE, Held N, Wright K. Raynaud's phenomenon of the nipple: a treatable cause of painful breastfeeding. *Pediatrics*. 2004; **113**: e360–4.

[2.11] Tranexamic acid (OTC)

Class: antifibrinolytic (inhibits the natural destruction of fibrin in clots)

Tablets: 500 mg

Dose: adults: 2 tablets 3 times a day, increasing to 4 times a day if necessary

Pack: 60

$t_{1/2}$:   2 h after intravenous (IV) injection (the duration of action of tablets will depend on the rate of absorption)

Side-effects: nausea, vomiting, diarrhoea (these often resolve if the dose is reduced), disturbance of colour vision (discontinue), rarely thrombotic events, convulsions, allergic skin reactions

Interactions: counteracts fibrinolytic drugs, such as streptokinase

Cautions: do not prescribe to anyone with a history of thromboembolic disease. Lower doses are required in renal impairment. There is no evidence of harm during breastfeeding

Selection: this is one of the few non-hormonal treatments for menorrhagia. Tranexamic acid causes a greater reduction of heavy menstrual bleeding and no increase in side-effects when compared with placebo or other medical therapies (NSAIDs, oral progestogens and etamsylate). It is probably underused because of misplaced fears about causing thrombosis. Long-term studies in Sweden have shown that the rate of thrombosis in women treated with tranexamic acid is comparable with the spontaneous backgound frequency

References

[No authors listed]. OTC tranexamic acid for heavy menstrual bleeding? *Drug Ther Bull*. 2011; **49**: 6–8.

Lethaby A, Farquhar C, Cooke I. Antifibrinolytics for heavy menstrual bleeding. *Cochrane Database Syst Rev*. 2000; **4**: CD000249.

Respiratory system

[3.1.1] Salbutamol (in an inhaler device to suit the patient)

Suiting the patient's needs and preferences is the priority, but good first choices are:
- Ventolin Evohaler® pressurised metered dose inhaler (+ spacer if needed)
- Salamol Easi-Breathe® breath-actuated inhaler
- Ventolin nebules®

Class:	β_2 adrenoceptor agonist (mimics the action of adrenaline at the β_2 receptors in the lungs)
Inhaler:	100 µg per dose
Nebules:	2.5 mg/2.5 mL, 5 mg/2.5 mL
Dose:	inhaler: adult 2 doses, child 1–2 doses
	nebulised: adult 5 mg, child 2.5 mg
	These doses can be repeated up to 4 times in a day if required, but follow the British Thoracic Society (BTS) asthma guidelines for appropriate treatment of persistent symptoms
Pack:	1 inhaler or 20 ampoules of nebuliser solution
$t_{1/2}$:	5 (4–6) h
Side-effects:	fine tremor (particularly hands), nervous tension, headache, tachycardia, hypokalaemia, disturbance of sleep and behaviour in children, allergic reactions including paradoxical bronchospasm with exacerbation of wheezing shortly after receiving a dose of salbutamol (discontinue and substitute ipratropium bromide)
Interactions:	high doses of salbutamol can cause dangerous hypokalaemia, particularly in combination with corticosteroids, diuretics, theophylline or hypoxia. Patients needing salbutamol should not be taking a beta-blocker (which has the opposite action), especially a non-selective one such as propranolol. BTS guideline puts it very clearly: 'β-blockers, including eye drops, are contraindicated in patients with asthma.' Salbutamol possibly reduces plasma concentration of digoxin
Cautions:	patients finding that salbutamol is not relieving their symptoms should seek medical advice and be treated according to the BTS guidelines. Increasing frequency of use of salbutamol suggests deteriorating asthma in need of anti-inflammatory treatment with inhaled or oral corticosteroids. Caution is needed when prescribing for patients with hyperthyroidism, ischaemic heart disease, arrhythmias, hypertension, or any predisposing factors to hypokalaemia
Selection:	short-acting β_2 adrenoceptor agonists are the first step in the management of asthma. Nebulisers offer no advantage over spacer devices for delivery, but some patients, who are either young children or frightened adults, find the nebuliser easier. Ideally, use a spacer device unless the attack is life-threatening, when a nebuliser driven by pressurised oxygen is better.

Easi-Breathe is the breath-actuated device most liked by patients, but is four times the cost of the standard inhaler when they contain salbutamol. If the patient uses a regular inhaled steroid, prescribe the same type of inhaler for their salbutamol. Match Ventolin Evohaler with Clenil Modulite and Salamol Easi-Breathe with Qvar Easi-Breathe. As the technique and dose of different inhalers varies between manufacturers, it is best to prescribe them by brand name

References

Cates CJ, Crilly JA, Rowe BH. Holding chambers (spacers) versus nebulisers for beta-agonist treatment of acute asthma. *Cochrane Database Syst Rev*. 2006; **2**: CD000052.

Direkwatanachai C, Teeratakulpisarn J, Suntornlohanakul S, *et al*. Comparison of salbutamol efficacy in children – via the metered-dose inhaler (MDI) with Volumatic spacer and via the dry powder inhaler, Easyhaler, with the nebuliser – in mild to moderate asthma exacerbation: a multicenter, randomized study. *Asian Pac J Allergy Immunol*. 2011; **29**: 25–33.

Lenney J, Innes JA, Crompton GK. Inappropriate inhaler use: assessment of use and patient preference of seven inhalation devices. *Respir Med*. 2000; **94**(5): 496–500.

Scottish Intercollegiate Guidelines Network (SIGN). *British Guideline on the Management of Asthma: SIGN guideline 101*. Edinburgh: Scottish Intercollegiate Guidelines Network; 2011. www.sign.ac.uk/pdf/sign101.pdf

[3.1.5] Volumatic® (OTC) and AeroChamber Plus® (OTC)

Class: spacer devices

Device: with mouthpiece or mask

Cautions: advise that the device should be washed no more often than once a month and is best left to dry in the air because wiping with a cloth creates a static electric charge on the plastic which can affect drug delivery. Replace the device every year

Selection: spacer devices reduce the need for coordination when using metered dose inhalers and slow the speed of the aerosol spray, improving the deposition of the drug in the lungs, with less being sprayed directly onto the back of the throat. However, a study in the elderly concluded that breath-activated and dry-powder inhalers were more likely to be used correctly than metered dose inhalers with large volume spacers. The *BNF* says that larger devices with one-way valves work better, but a systematic review of inhaler devices showed no difference in efficacy, and the smaller AeroChamber Plus may be much more convenient for some patients. Children aged 2–7 years need two normal breaths to empty the AeroChamber Plus and three to empty the Volumatic. AeroChamber Plus has an adapter to suit all pressurised MDIs. Volumatic is design to fit the Ventolin Evohaler, but also works with Clenil Modulite, Flixotide, Seretide and Serevent

References

Jones V, Fernandez C, Diggory P. A comparison of large volume spacer, breath-activated and dry powder inhalers in older people. *Age Ageing.* 1999; **28**(5): 481–4.

Mazhar SH, Chrystyn H. Salbutamol relative lung and systemic bioavailability of large and small spacers. *J Pharm Pharmacol.* 2008; **60**: 1609–13.

NHS Centre for Reviews and Dissemination. Inhaler devices for the management of asthma and COPD. *Eff Health Care.* 2003; **8**(1): 1–12.

Schultz A, Le Souef TJ, Venter A, *et al.* Aerosol inhalation from spacers and valved holding chambers requires few tidal breaths for children. *Pediatrics.* 2010; **126**: e1493–8.

[3.1.5] Peak flow meter (OTC)

Class:	disease-monitoring device
Device:	standard range for adults and children, low range for adults who can only manage peak flows less than 400 L/minute or children
Cautions:	children under 5 years of age cannot reliably use a peak flow meter, and older ones cannot be expected to keep an acute record of their readings. From 2004, EU meters produce different readings from the previous type; for a conversion calculator and normal ranges, see www.peakflow.com
Selection:	all peak flow meters available on an NHS prescription conform to a European standard, so it does not matter which one you choose. In addition to mechanical devices, a small digital device (Piko-1) is available at slightly higher cost. An asthma management plan, whereby the patient knows what to do if their condition starts to deteriorate, is what matters, rather than whether it is based on symptoms or peak flow readings

References

Kamps AW, Roorda RJ, Brand PL. Peak flow diaries in childhood asthma are unreliable. *Thorax*. 2001; **56**(3): 180–2.

Powell H, Gibson PG. Options for self-management education for adults with asthma. *Cochrane Database Syst Rev*. 2003; **1**: CD004107.

[3.2] Beclometasone (in an inhaler device to suit the patient)

Good first choices are:

- Clenil Modulite® pressurised metered dose inhaler (+ spacer if needed)
- Qvar Easi-Breathe® breath-actuated inhaler

Class:	inhaled corticosteroid
Inhaler:	50, 100 and, in Clenil Modulite only, 200, 250 µg per dose
Dose:	note the equipotent dose of Qvar is about half that of Clenil Modulite, so it is essential to prescribe CFC-free beclometasone by brand name
	see text on acute asthma, 50–800 µg/day
Pack:	200-dose inhaler
$t_{1/2}$**:**	0.5–2.7 h. What matters clinically is that the time to maximum effect of the first dose is 2–8 h by whatever route the corticosteroid is administered. Maximum effect of repeated doses of inhaled beclometasone may not be achieved for 3–7 days
Side-effects:	may precipitate oral thrush (in which case use a spacer and rinse mouth after use), rarely paradoxical bronchospasm, glaucoma, cataracts
Interactions:	there are some case reports of accumulation of inhaled corticosteroid from interactions with itraconazole and ritonavir (*see* CYP450 under 'Cautions')
Cautions:	tuberculosis (quiescent disease may be reactivated), high doses may induce adrenal suppression – patients taking above the normal maximum licensed dose (usually taken to mean 800 µg/day; under 12 years 400 µg/day) for prolonged periods should be issued with a steroid card, children's height monitored and adults considered for monitoring of bone mineral density. The MRHA has suggested that patients taking normal doses of inhaled corticosteroid would also need a steroid card and monitoring if they were taking a medication that inhibited the CYP450 enzyme system (see http://medicine.iupui.edu/clinpharm/ddis/table.aspx), but such caution has not been widely adopted
Selection:	at equipotent doses, the type of corticosteroid makes no difference to its effectiveness. This is the reason that national guidelines recommend prescribing the cheapest. The delivery system should suit the patient. As the technique and dose of different inhalers varies between manufacturers, it is best to prescribe them by brand name

References

Bolland MJ, Bagg W, Thomas MG, *et al*. Cushing's syndrome due to interaction between inhaled corticosteroids and itraconazole. *Ann Pharmacother*. 2004; **38**: 46–9.

Iwasaki E, Baba M. [Pharmacokinetics and pharmacodynamics of hydrocortisone in asthmatic children] [Japanese]. *Arerugi*. 1993; **42**(10): 1555–62.

Medicines and Healthcare products Regulatory Agency and Commission on Human Medicines. High dose inhaled steroids: new advice on supply of steroid treatment cards. *Current Problems in Pharmacovigilance*. 2006; **31**: 5.

[3.4.1] Cetirizine (OTC)

Class:	histamine (H_1) receptor blocker
Tablets:	10 mg
Liquid:	5 mg/5 mL
Dose:	adults and children over 6 years: 10 mg once a day *or* 5 mg twice a day
	children 2–6 years: 5 mg once a day *or* 2.5 mg twice a day
Pack:	30 tablets, or 200 mL
$t_{1/2}$:	10 h (3–6 h in children)
Side-effects:	dry mouth, headache, incidence of sedation is low, but it is still worth warning drivers to be alert to the slight possibility of drowsiness or dizziness
Interactions:	theoretical antagonism of betahistine
Cautions:	renal disease, myasthenia gravis, poor dental hygiene (dry mouth increases risk of caries). Cetirizine is generally regarded as safe in pregnancy and breastfeeding, although the manufacturers advise caution
Selection:	cetirizine is available OTC. The cost for 1 month's supply is less than a prescription charge. The duration of the antihistaminic effect is much longer than would be predicted from the serum elimination half-life, but if the effect of the drug does not last through the day, or if symptoms are troublesome in the evening or at night, use twice-daily dosing. This is more likely for children because they eliminate the drug faster than adults. All non-sedating antihistamines have a low risk of causing drowsiness, but cetirizine has a slightly higher risk than loratadine. Cetirizine is less expensive than fexofenadine

References

Mann RD, Pearce GL, Dunn N, *et al*. Sedation with 'non-sedating' antihistamines: four prescription-event monitoring studies in general practice. *BMJ*. 2000; **320**: 1184–7.

NHS Choices. *Can I Take Hay Fever Medicine During Pregnancy?* 2011. Available at: www.nhs.uk/chq/Pages/home.aspx

Pariente-Khayat A, Rey E, Dubois MC, *et al*. Pharmacokinetics of cetirizine in 2- to 6-year-old children. *Int J Clin Pharmacol Ther*. 1995; **33**: 340–4.

Spicak V, Dab I, Hulhoven R, *et al*. Pharmacokinetics and pharmacodynamics of cetirizine in infants and toddlers. *Clin Pharmacol Ther*. 1997; **61**: 325–30.

UKMi Central. *Drugs in Lactation*. 2011. Available at: www.ukmicentral.nhs.uk/drugpreg/antihistamines.asp (accessed 26 August 2011).

[3.4.1] Loratadine (OTC)

Class:	histamine (H_1) receptor blocker
Tablets:	10 mg
Liquid:	5 mg/5 mL
Dose:	adults and children over 6 years: 10 mg once a day
	children 2–6 years: 5 mg once a day
Pack:	30 tablets; 100 mL liquid
$t_{1/2}$:	15 h, but the active metabolite is longer at 18–37 h
Side-effects:	headache, nervousness in children occasionally, incidence of sedation is low but it is still worth warning drivers to be alert to the slight possibility of drowsiness or dizziness
Interactions:	theoretical antagonism of betahistine
Cautions:	loratadine is generally regarded as safe in pregnancy and breastfeeding, although the manufacturers do not recommend this
Selection:	all non-sedating antihistamines have a low risk of causing drowsiness, but loratadine has a very low risk and may be more suitable for people who have a safety-critical occupation. Loratadine is approximately six times less expensive than its active metabolite, desloratadine

References

NHS Choices. *Can I Take Hay Fever Medicine During Pregnancy?* 2011. Available at: www.nhs.uk/chq/Pages/935.aspx?categoryid=73&subcategoryid=107

Ramaekers JG, Vermeeren A. All antihistamines cross blood-brain barrier. *BMJ*. 2000; **321**: 572.

UKMi Central. *Drugs in Lactation*. 2011. Available at: www.ukmicentral.nhs.uk/drugpreg/antihistamines.asp (accessed 26 August 2011).

[3.4.1] Chlorphenamine (OTC)

Class:	histamine (H$_1$) receptor blocker
Tablets:	4 mg
Liquid:	2 mg/5 mL
Dose:	although the doses below are quoted in the *BNF*, the long half-life of chlorphenamine means that a single dose can suffice in most individuals
	adults and children over 12 years: 4 mg every 4–6 h, maximum 24 mg daily
	children 6–12 years: 2 mg every 4–6 h, maximum 12 mg daily
	2–6 years: 1 mg every 4–6 h, maximum 6 mg daily
	1 month–2 years: 1 mg twice a day
Pack:	28 tablets; 150 mL liquid
$t_{1/2}$:	18 (12–34) h, with considerable variability between individuals
Side-effects:	drowsiness may affect performance of skilled tasks, e.g. driving; headache, psychomotor impairment, dry mouth, blurred vision, urinary retention and gastrointestinal disturbances; occasionally allergic reactions such as rashes or photosensitivity; rarely paradoxical stimulation. Children and elderly people are particularly susceptible to side-effects
Interactions:	sedatives (including alcohol), MAOI and tricyclic antidepressants
Cautions:	prostatic hypertrophy, urinary retention, glaucoma, hepatic or renal disease, epilepsy. Allow enough time for the effects to wear off before the patient returns to any activity that could be dangerous under sedation
Selection:	chlorphenamine is useful when sedation is helpful, such as disruption of sleep caused by skin irritation or cough. The sedative effect is mediated by blocking histamine H$_1$ receptors in the brain, which is why loratadine and cetirizine, which do not cross the blood-brain barrier so much, are less likely to cause this effect

References

Sen A, Akin A, Craft KJ, *et al*. First-generation H$_1$ antihistamines found in pilot fatalities of civil aviation accidents, 1990–2005. *Aviat Space Environ Med*. 2007; 78: 514–22.

Simons KJ, Martin TJ, Watson WT, *et al*. Pharmacokinetics and pharmacodynamics of terfenadine and chlorpheniramine in the elderly. *J Allergy Clini Immunol*. 1990; 85(3): 540–7.

[3.8] Menthol and eucalyptus (OTC)

Class: aromatic inhalation

Liquid: race- or levo-menthol 2 g, eucalyptus oil 10 mL, light magnesium carbonate 7 g, water to 100 mL

Dose: add 1 teaspoonful to a pint of hot water and inhale vapour

Pack: 100 mL

Side-effects: only scalds from spilling the water

Interactions: none

Cautions: use hot, not boiling water. May induce apnoea in infants less than 3 months

Selection: the ingredients may not have any direct effect but encourage the inhalation of water vapour, which can be soothing in bronchitis or sinusitis, and may also have a useful placebo action. Inhaler devices which may reduce the risk of scalding are available for about £7

Reference

Kenia P, Houghton T, Beardsmore C. Does inhaling menthol affect nasal patency or cough? *Pediatr Pulmonol.* 2008; **43**: 532–7.

[3.9.2] Simple linctus (OTC)

Class:	demulcent cough linctus
Linctus:	adults: citric acid monohydrate 2.5% in a suitable vehicle with anise flavour (sugar-free available)
	children: citric acid monohydrate 0.625% in a suitable vehicle with anise flavour (sugar-free available)
Dose:	adults and children over 12 years: 5 mL of adult linctus 4 times daily
	children 6–12 years: 5–10 mL of paediatric linctus 4 times daily
Pack:	200 mL
Side-effects:	none
Interactions:	none
Cautions:	none
Selection:	before prescribing, ask yourself if it is appropriate to try to reduce the coughing. For children and adolescents, honey appears to be just as good. Chocolate may be even better, but clinical trials are needed: any volunteers? Adults may be distressed by a dry, unproductive cough. Simple linctus contains soothing substances that may help patients to tolerate a dry irritating cough without any risk of side-effects. Note this is quite different from expectorants, which claim to promote the coughing up of sputum. There is no evidence of effectiveness of any OTC cough linctus. Quite often, patients attend because of a persisting cough for which they are taking an expectorant type of cough medicine inappropriately; all that is required is to stop the expectorant. In children, coughing is usually helpful, but if necessary a sedative antihistamine is more effective at providing some rest at night than a linctus

References

Medicines and Healthcare products Regulatory Agency. *Children's Over-the-Counter Cough and Cold Medicines: new advice.* 2011. www.mhra.gov.uk/Safetyinformation/Safetywarnings alertsandrecalls/Safetywarningsandmessagesformedicines/CON038908

Paul IM, Beiler J, McMonagle A, *et al.* Effect of honey, dextromethorphan, and no treatment on nocturnal cough and sleep quality for coughing children and their parents. *Arch Pediatr Adolesc Med.* 2007; **161**: 1140–6.

Schroeder K, Fahey T. Should we advise parents to administer over the counter cough medicines for acute cough? Systematic review of randomised controlled trials. *Arch Dis Child.* 2002; **86**: 170–5.

Schroeder K, Fahey T. Systematic review of randomised controlled trials of over the counter cough medicines for acute cough in adults. *BMJ.* 2002; **324**: 329–31.

Usmani OS, Belvisi MG, Patel HJ, *et al.* Theobromine inhibits sensory nerve activation and cough. *FASEB J.* 2005; **19**(2): 231–3.

Nervous system

[4.1.1] Temazepam (CD)

Class:	benzodiazepine hypnotic
Tablets:	10 mg
Dose:	1 alternate nights
Pack:	28, but limit prescriptions to 7 tablets
$t_{1/2}$:	men: 12 (7–15) h; women: 17 h; overall range: 8–38 h
Side-effects:	drowsiness and light-headedness the next day; confusion, paradoxical agitation and ataxia (especially in the elderly); addiction after long-term use
Interactions:	enhanced sedation with other sedatives (including alcohol), opiates, tricyclic antidepressants, antihistamines, antipsychotics, disulfram, lofexidine, baclofen, tizanidine, cimetidine
Cautions:	potentially addictive, may cause daytime drowsiness the following day and affect driving, increases the effect of alcohol. Do not use in those with chronic chest disease, liver or renal disease, or in pregnancy or breastfeeding
Selection:	hypnotics are occasionally very useful for short-term relief of insomnia – usually related to psychological stress, but are not suitable for long-term use because of the risk of addiction and the fact that there is often a better, non-pharmacological solution to the problem. Temazepam has the advantage of being one of the shorter-acting hypnotics and is therefore less likely to cause drowsiness the next day, although it is not free of this risk, particularly in women. Be careful to warn patients that it may impair their driving ability the next morning. Other hypnotics may have a much longer duration of action (e.g. diazepam), causing persisting drowsiness, or a shorter duration (e.g. Z-drugs) that risk causing a withdrawal effect of early morning insomnia. Age does not seem to affect the duration of action of the drug, but the elderly are more susceptible to side-effects. Tolerance does not appear to be a problem. Amendments to the Misuse of Drugs Regulations came into force in July 2006, limiting the validity of a temazepam prescription to 28 days, instead of the normal 6 months

References

Divoll M, Greenblatt DJ, Harmatz JS, *et al*. Effect of age and gender on disposition of temazepam. *J Pharm Sci*. 1981; **70**(10): 1104–7.

Van Steveninck AL, Wallnofer AE, Schoemaker RC, *et al*. A study of the effects of long-term use on individual sensitivity to temazepam and lorazepam in a clinical population. *Br J Clin Pharmacol*. 1997; **44**(3): 267–75.

[4.6] Prochlorperazine (buccal tablets OTC to people over 18, limited amount)

Class:	phenothiazine-type antiemetic
Tablets:	5 mg
Buccal tablets:	3 mg
Liquid:	5 mg/5 mL
Dose:	adults only, tablets or liquid
	labyrinthitis: 5 mg 3 times daily initially
	acute nausea/vomiting: 20 mg initially, 10 mg after 2 h
	prevention of nausea/vomiting: 5–10 mg three times daily
	buccal tablets: 1 or 2 tablets twice a day, place high between lip and gum and leave to dissolve
	(buccal 3 mg twice daily is equivalent to an oral dose of 5 mg 3 times daily)
Pack:	28 tablets; 8 (OTC) or 50 (subdivided into 5 × 10) buccal tablets; 100 mL liquid
$t_{1/2}$:	8 (6–10) h
Side-effects:	for a full list, see the *BNF* under chlorpromazine, but in practice the only common one is drowsiness, and very occasionally severe dystonic reactions (see below)
Interactions:	enhanced sedation with other sedatives (including alcohol), desferrioxamine, dopaminergic drugs in Parkinson's disease (e.g. levodopa), lithium
Cautions:	may cause severe dystonic reactions (abnormal face and body movements). This is rare, but more common in teenagers and young adults (acute 'oculogyric' reactions); the elderly (delayed Parkinsonian-type reactions); and the risk may be exacerbated by a concurrent viral illness. It is therefore wise to avoid prescribing prochlorperazine for these groups
Selection:	prochlorperazine is useful when sedation is helpful in addition to an antiemetic action. Often the distress of feeling nauseous is a major part of the problem, and a degree of sedation is welcome. As the end of the drug name implies, this belongs to the phenothiazine group of drugs, other members of which are used as antipsychotics. Thus it is no surprise that prochlorperazine is liable to give rise to central nervous system side-effects, and this is what limits its use

References

Hessell PG, Lloyd-Jones JG, Muir NC, *et al.* A comparison of the availability of prochlorperazine following i.m., buccal and oral administration. *Int J Pharmaceutics.* 1989; **52**: 159–64.

Isah AO, Rawlins MD, Bateman DN. Clinical pharmacology of prochlorperazine in healthy young males. *Br J Clin Pharmacol.* 1991; **32**(6): 677–84.

Schumock GT, Martinez E. Acute oculogyric crisis after administration of prochlorperazine. *South Med J.* 1991; **84**(3): 407–8.

[4.6] Domperidone (OTC, limited amount; promoted for dyspepsia rather than nausea)

Class:	dopamine (D_2) receptor blocker
Tablets:	10 mg
Liquid:	5 mg/5 mL
Suppositories:	30 mg
Dose:	adults and children over 35 kg body weight:
	oral: 10–20 mg up to 4 times a day
	rectal: 60 mg twice daily
Pack:	30 tablets; 200 mL liquid; 10 suppositories
$t_{1/2}$:	7 h
Side-effects:	raised prolactin concentrations (possible breast tissue enlargement and leakage of milk from the nipples); occasionally reduced libido and, very rarely, acute dystonic reactions. Recently, there has been concern raised over an increased risk of sudden cardiac death with daily doses over 30 mg
Interactions:	antagonised by opioid analgesics, accelerated absorption of paracetamol
Cautions:	avoid if the patient has a known long QTc interval on ECG, liver disease, pregnancy, prolactinoma; reduce dose frequency in renal impairment to once or twice daily depending on the severity of the impairment
Selection:	because domperidone does not cross the blood-brain barrier, the acute dystonic reactions seen with metoclopramide and prochlorperazine are much less likely to occur. It blocks peripheral D_2 receptors, including those in the chemoreceptor trigger zone. It is a logical choice to minimise drug-induced nausea (e.g. associated with post-coital contraception) when sedation is not required and minimising the risk of side-effects is paramount

References

Barone JA. Domperidone: a peripherally acting dopamine2-receptor antagonist [review]. *Ann Pharmacother*. 1999; **33**(4): 429–40.

Van Noord C, Dieleman JP, Van Herpen G, *et al*. Domperidone and ventricular arrhythmia or sudden cardiac death: a population-based case-control study in the Netherlands. *Drug Saf*. 2010; **33**: 1003–14.

www.qtdrugs.org

[4.7.1] Aspirin (OTC)

Class:	antiplatelet agent/analgesic
Tablets:	75 mg, 300 mg (dispersible)
Dose:	adults, ideally taken with or after food
	anti-thrombotic: 75–300 mg daily (usually 75 mg daily for long-term use, and 300 mg as the first dose for acute coronary syndrome)
	acute migraine: 900 mg dispersible as soon as possible once the symptoms of an acute migraine are recognized
Pack:	100
$t_{1/2}$:	2–3 h, but the clinical effect of 300 mg lasts 24 h and the haematological effect lasts 10 days
Side-effects:	high incidence of gastrointestinal irritation with slight asymptomatic blood loss, increased bleeding time, bronchospasm and skin reactions in hypersensitive patients
Interactions:	important interaction with **warfarin**, avoid co-prescribing with NSAIDs or **methotrexate**, increased risk of bleeding with SSRI antidepressants, clopidogrel or corticosteroids
Cautions:	*not for use by children under 16*, allergy, peptic ulcer, gout, pregnancy, breastfeeding, asthma (a small proportion of asthmatic patients find that aspirin worsens their symptoms; occasionally this can be severe)
Selection:	antithrombotic action: aspirin disables an enzyme essential to the action of platelets sticking together. As platelets have no cell nucleus, they never recover this ability, but 10% of the platelet population are replaced daily. A single dose of 300 mg inhibits all platelets; 75 mg inhibits about 30% and can be used to maintain antiplatelet action. Platelet function is restored to near normal 24 h after stopping aspirin by the 10% of newly formed platelets, so missing a dose or two can cause the protection against strokes and heart attacks to be lost. Acute migraine can be treated effectively with aspirin. The dispersible tablets are preferred because some patients will have difficulty swallowing if nauseous. Inhibition of gastric movements may delay the absorption of solid tablets, but the average time delay is only 10 minutes

References

Furukawa K, Hitoshi O. Inhibition of platelet aggregation with aspirin falls quickly at 1 day after discontinuation and vanished after 3 days. *J Thorac Cardiovasc Surg.* 2004; **127**: 1814–15.

Lampl C, Voelker M, Diener HC. Efficacy and safety of 1,000 mg effervescent aspirin: individual patient data meta-analysis of three trials in migraine headache and migraine accompanying symptoms. *J Neurol.* 2007; **254**: 705–12.

[4.7.1] Paracetamol (OTC)

Class:	non-opioid analgesic
Tablets:	500 mg
Soluble tablets:	120 mg (paediatric), 500 mg
Liquid:	120 mg/5 mL, 250 mg/5 mL
Suppositories:	60, 125, 250, 500 mg (expensive)
Dose:	all up to 4 times a day, by mouth or by rectum
	adults > 50 kg: 1000 mg
	adults < 50 kg: 500 mg
	note: the doses for children were updated in 2011
	children 10–18 years: 500 mg
	8–10 years: 375 mg
	6–8 years: 250 mg
	4–6 years: 240 mg
	2–4 years: 180 mg
	6 months–2 years: 120 mg
	3–6 months: 60 mg
Pack:	16, 32 tablets; 100, 150, 200, 500 mL liquid; 10 suppositories
$t_{1/2}$:	2 (1–3) h
Side-effects:	overdose is the only serious problem
Interactions:	prolonged regular use possibly enhances warfarin, colestyramine reduces absorption of paracetamol, whereas metoclopramide, domperidone and sodium bicarbonate can accelerate it
Cautions:	overdosage with paracetamol is particularly dangerous as it may cause hepatic damage which is sometimes not apparent for 4–6 days. Legislation to limit the pack sizes available over the counter has reduced the number of deaths and large overdoses, so prescribing a limited supply for acute self-limiting conditions may help achieve the same aim. Those with pre-existing liver disease or taking enzyme-inducing drugs (including alcohol) makes the potential for toxic effects greater. Malnourished individuals without liver disease are also at higher risk, so for those weighing under 50 kg limit the daily dose to 2 g. Although paracetamol is often given to babies under 3 months of age to prevent or treat post-immunisation pyrexia, the Department of Health stated in 2011: 'It is not recommended that these drugs are used routinely to prevent fever following vaccination, as there is some evidence that prophylactic administration of antipyretic drugs around the time of vaccination may lower antibody responses to some vaccines.' Neonates absorb and eliminate paracetamol differently to older children and adults, but toxic effects from paracetamol are most unlikely. Suppositories are expensive, costing about £1 each
Selection:	paracetamol is virtually free of side-effects when taken in the normal dose range. This makes it a very useful analgesic. It is commonly used to treat

fever, but consider first if it is necessary to interfere with a normal biological response to infection and second, whether the more effective ibuprofen would be a better option for this purpose

References

Arana A, Morton NS, Hansen TG. Treatment with paracetamol in infants [review]. *Act Anaesth Scand*. 2001; **45**(1): 20–9.

Claridge LC, Eksteen B, Smith A, Shah T, Holt AP. Acute liver failure after administration of paracetamol at the maximum recommended daily dose in adults. *BMJ*. 2010; **341**: c6764.

Department of Health. *Update to Immunisation Against Infectious Disease*. 2011. Available at: www.dh.gov.uk

Isbister GK, Bucens IK, Whyte IM. Paracetamol overdose in a preterm neonate. *Arch Dis Child*. 2001; **85**(1): F70–2.

Harnden A. Antipyretic treatment for feverish young children in primary care. *BMJ*. 2008; **337**: a1409.

Hawton K, Simkin S, Deeks J, *et al*. UK legislation on analgesic packs: before and after study of long term effect on poisonings. *BMJ*. 2004; **329**: 1076–9.

Hay AD, Costelloe C, Redmond NM, *et al*. Paracetamol plus ibuprofen for the treatment of fever in children (PITCH): randomised controlled trial. *BMJ*. 2008; **337**: a1302.

Medicines and Healthcare products Regulatory Agency. *More Exact Paracetamol Dosing for Children to be Introduced*. Press Release. London: MHRA; 6 June 2011. Available at: www.mhra.gov.uk/NewsCentre/Pressreleases/CON120251 (accessed 2 January 2012).

Prymula R, Siegrist C, Chiblek R. Effect of prophylactic paracetamol administration at time of vaccination on febrile reactions and antibody responses in children: two open-label, randomised controlled trials. *Lancet*. 2009; **374**: 1339–50.

Wan Y. *BMJ Lesson of the Week: Acute liver failure after administration of paracetamol at recommended daily dose. Summary*. National electronic Library for Medicines; 2010. www.nelm.nhs.uk//en/NeLM-Area/News/2010---December/03/BMJ-lesson-of-the-week-Acute-liver-failure-after-administration-of-paracetamol-at-maximum-recommended-daily-dose/ (accessed 28 November 2011).

[4.7.2] Codeine phosphate

Class:	opioid analgesic
Tablets:	30 mg
Dose:	adults: 30 mg when required up to 4-hourly
Pack:	28
$t_{1/2}$:	3 h
Side-effects:	constipation, nausea, dependence, may cause drowsiness, respiratory depression, hypotension, difficulty with micturition and a variety of rare side-effects listed in the *BNF* under morphine
Interactions:	sedatives (including alcohol), MAOI-type antidepressants, cimetidine, reduced action of domperidone and metoclopramide on the gut
Cautions:	avoid in significant respiratory, renal or liver (including biliary) disease, or after a head injury, breastfeeding or in the third trimester of pregnancy; may exacerbate urinary obstructive symptoms, or confusion in elderly or debilitated. To take this drug abroad, patients may require a letter from their doctor stating that it is a necessary medication
Selection:	codeine is effective at improving the analgesia provided by paracetamol, but only if it is taken in an adequate dose. The best dose to balance effectiveness against side-effects is 30 mg. Fixed combination tablets containing paracetamol/codeine in ratios of 500/8 mg or 500/30 mg make it impossible to achieve the best dose of each analgesic. The 500/15 mg combination is better, but more expensive, and still deprives the patient of the options provided by using the drugs separately. Prescribing codeine separately gives the patient freedom to match the analgesic they take to the degree of pain: paracetamol alone for mild pain, codeine alone for more moderate, or both for more severe pain. Minimising the need to take the codeine with every dose minimises the side-effects. Dihydrocodeine offers no advantages over codeine. The codeine group of analgesics can increase biliary spasm, so are not suitable to relieve biliary colic. NSAIDs (such as ibuprofen) are preferable for inflammatory conditions or dental pain. There is considerable variation in the proportion of codeine metabolised into morphine, particularly in women, so codeine is not suitable for use in breastfeeding when the variable amount of morphine can pose a risk to the baby

References

MacDonald N, MacLeod SM. Has the time come to phase out codeine? *CMAJ*. 2010; **182**: 1825.

Mehlisch D, Frakes L, Cavaliere MB, *et al*. Double-blind parallel comparison of single oral doses of ketoprofen, codeine, and placebo in patients with moderate to severe dental pain. *J Clin Pharmacol*. 1984; **24**: 486–92.

Moore A, Collins S, Carroll D, *et al*. Paracetamol with and without codeine in acute pain: a quantitative systematic review. *Pain*. 1997; **70**(2–3): 193–201.

[4.7.4.] Sumatriptan (OTC)

Class:	serotonin ($5HT_{1D}$) receptor agonist
Tablets:	50, 100 mg
Dose:	adults: 50 mg is the usual dose for acute migraine, but individual response varies and 25 mg may suffice for some, while others need 100 mg. The dose may be repeated after 2 h if migraine recurs. Maximum of 300 mg in 24 h
	children: not licensed but occasionally used (see *BNFC* for details) despite a number of placebo-controlled clinical studies showing no benefit
Pack:	6 tablets
$t_{1/2}$**:**	2 h
Side-effects:	*common:* tingling and warmth, pain, heaviness or pressure sensations (including the chest), flushing, dizziness, weakness, myalgia (that can include aching mimicking neck stiffness), fatigue, transient increase in blood pressure, dyspnoea; occasionally nausea, vomiting, allergic reactions, seizures, movement disorders, visual changes, arrhythmias, angina and myocardial infarction, diarrhoea, ischaemic colitis, hypotension, anxiety, Raynaud's syndrome, sweating
Interactions:	most antidepressants: selective serotonin reuptake inhibitors (e.g. fluoxetine), duloxetine, venlafaxine, monoamine oxidase inhibitors, St John's wort; selegiline, ergotamine, methysergide
Cautions:	avoid in vascular disease: ischaemic heart disease (including any history of a previous myocardial infarction), cerebrovascular disease (including any history of a previous stroke or transient ischaemic attack), poorly controlled hypertension, peripheral vascular disease; caution if the risk of possible ischaemic heart disease is high
Selection:	several anti-migraine drugs of this type are now available, but sumatriptan was the first in the UK. Thus it has the longest history of use, leading to low cost of the generic product and OTC availability for people who have a diagnosis of migraine. Avoid prescribing it by brand name as this would increase the cost 25-fold for no good reason. Alternative 'triptans' have a similar mode of action, but vary in their efficacy and side-effect profile. It is important to choose one that suits the patient. About 40% of migraine sufferers will not gain relief from sumatriptan within 2 h. Efficacy may be improved by co-prescribing naproxen. The main problem with sumatriptan is the frequency of side-effects. If this proves to be the limiting factor, consider naratriptan, which has a lower frequency of side-effects and a slower action

References

Belvis R, Pagonabarraga J, Kulisevsky J. Individual triptan selection in migraine attack therapy. *Recent Pat CNS Drug Discov.* 2009; **4**: 70–81.

Evans EW, Lorber KC. Use of 5-HT1 agonists in pregnancy. *Ann Pharmacother.* 2008; **42**: 543–9.

Ferrari MD, Roon KI, Lipton RB, *et al*. Oral triptans (serotonin 5-HT (1B/1D) agonists) in acute migraine treatment: a meta-analysis of 53 trials. *Lancet*. 2001; **358**: 1668–75.

Saper JR. What matters is not the differences between triptans, but the differences between patients [letter; comment]. *Arch Neurol-Chicago*. 2001; **58**: 1481–2.

Infections

[5.1.1] Phenoxymethylpenicillin

Class:	narrow-spectrum, bactericidal antibiotic
Tablets:	250 mg
Liquid:	125 mg/5 mL, 250 mg/5 mL
Dose:	all 4 times a day, on an empty stomach
	adults: 500 mg, increased to 1 g in severe infections
	children: 6–12 years 250 mg
	1–6 years 125 mg
	1 month–1 year 62.5 mg
	all paediatric doses can be increased up to 12.5 mg/kg in severe infections
Pack:	28 tablets – but the usual prescription for streptococcal tonsillitis in adults is 80 tablets; 100 mL liquid – usually 200 mL required. The liquid has a very short shelf life
$t_{1/2}$:	45 (30–60) minutes
Side-effects:	hypersensitivity reactions including urticaria, fever, joint pains, rashes, angio-oedema, and in severe cases anaphylaxis; interstitial nephritis; antibiotic-associated diarrhoea, reduction in platelet, white or red blood cell counts, increased risk of bleeding, rarely convulsions
Interactions:	does not affect oral contraceptives or warfarin
Cautions:	penicillin allergy, lower doses may be needed in severe renal impairment (eGFR < 15)
Selection:	phenoxymethylpenicillin is useful for treating streptococcal tonsillitis, but the absorption is too variable for the antibiotic to be reliably used for serious infections or those needing fast onset of action. Note the adult dose recommended by authorities in the UK starts at 500 mg 4 times daily. Otherwise the variable absorption can result in sub-therapeutic blood level, leading to treatment failure and the risk of developing resistant bacteria. Prescribing a 10-day course may reduce the chance of recurrence of the infection. The main problem when prescribing for children is the poor compliance – try tasting the suspension and you will find out why. Amoxicillin is a suitable alternative for treating streptococcal infections in children

References

Gopichand I, Williams GD, Medendorp SV, *et al*. Randomized, single-blinded comparative study of the efficacy of amoxicillin (40 mg/kg/day) versus standard-dose penicillin V in the treatment of group A streptococcal pharyngitis in children. *Clin Pediatr.* 1998; **37**: 341–6.

Hoppe JE, Blumenstock G, Grotz W, *et al*. Compliance of German pediatric patients with oral antibiotic therapy: results of a nationwide survey. *Pediatr Infect Dis J*. 1999; **18**: 1085–91.

Joint Formulary Committee. *British National Formulary.* London: BMJ Group and Pharmaceutical Press. 2011; **61**: 334.

Schwartz RH, Wientzen RL Jr, Pedreira F, *et al*. Penicillin V for group A streptococcal pharyngotonsillitis. A randomized trial of seven vs ten days' therapy. *JAMA*. 1981; **246**: 1790–5.

[5.1.1.2] Flucloxacillin

Class:	β-lactamase-resistant narrow-spectrum bactericidal antibacterial
Capsules:	250, 500 mg
Oral solution:	125 mg/5 mL, 250 mg/5 mL
Dose:	all 4 times a day, 1 h before food or on an empty stomach; doses may be doubled in severe infection
	adults and children over 10 years: usually 250 mg, increased to 500 mg for 10–14 days for cellulitis and 2 weeks for mastitis during lactation
	children 2–10 years: 125 mg
	1 month–2 years: 62.5 mg
Pack:	28 capsules, 100 mL liquid
$t_{1/2}$:	1 h
Side-effects:	*see* phenoxymethylpenicillin, page 189; rarely hepatitis, cholestatic jaundice which can develop several weeks after the course (the risk is greater for courses longer than 2 weeks and for older patients)
Interactions:	does not affect oral contraceptives or warfarin
Cautions:	penicillin allergy, porphyria, children may not like the taste — co-amoxiclav is then an alternative, though broader spectrum
Selection:	this is the standard treatment against staphylococcal infections

References

Matsui D, Barron A, Rieder MJ. Assessment of the palatability of antistaphylococcal antibiotics in pediatric volunteers. *Ann Pharmacother*. 1996; **30**: 586–8.

Miros M, Kerlin P, Walker N, *et al*. Flucloxacillin induced delayed cholestatic hepatitis. *Austral NZ J Med*. 1990; **20**(3): 251–3.

[5.1.1.3] Amoxicillin

Class:	broad-spectrum, bactericidal antibacterial
Capsules:	250, 500 mg
Liquid:	125 mg/1.25 mL, 125 mg/5 mL, 250 mg/5 mL
Sachets:	3 g
Dose:	all 3 times a day, doubled in severe infection

adults: 500 mg

children 5–18 years: 250 mg

1–5 years: 125 mg

1 month–1 year: 62.5 mg

for otitis media: adults and children over 75 kg, 1 g 3 times a day; children under 75 kg, 40 mg/kg daily in 3 divided doses

for dental abscess: adults, 3 g repeated once after 8 h

for urinary tract infections known to be sensitive to amoxicillin: adults, 3 g repeated once after 10–12 h

note: recommended doses of amoxicillin vary between difference authoritative references. The above doses are appropriate for the likely infections presenting to a clinic providing urgent access in primary care

Pack:	21; 100 mL; 20 mL of paediatric liquid 125 mg/1.25 mL
$t_{1/2}$:	1 h
Side-effects:	nausea, diarrhoea, rashes, allergic reactions; also *see* phenoxymethylpenicillin, page 189
Interactions:	warfarin effect may be altered, **no** reduction in efficacy of oral contraceptives
Cautions:	allergy, glandular fever (may cause rash), lower doses may be needed in severe renal impairment (eGFR < 15 mL/min/1.73 m²)
Selection:	amoxicillin is a broad-spectrum antibacterial suitable for treating a wide variety of infections. It is better absorbed than ampicillin and not affected by food. The paediatric liquid (125 mg/1.25 mL) is available in peach, strawberry and lemon flavours; the standard liquid is banana-flavoured. This choice may help concordance, but we have found no evidence for this, which is surprising given the 29% non-concordance reported for amoxicillin liquids taken by children. If compliance is an issue, then twice-daily dosing providing the same daily dose is an option. The cost of the paediatric liquid (125 mg/1.25 mL) is approximately three times more than the standard liquid form

References

Christian-Kopp S, Sinha M, Rosenberg DI, *et al*. Antibiotic dosing for acute otitis media in children: a weighty issue. *Pediatr Emerg Care*. 2010; **26**: 19–25.

Faculty of Sexual & Reproductive Healthcare. *Drug Interactions with Hormonal Contraception*. 2011. Available at: www.fsrh.org

Hoppe JE, Wahrenberger C. Compliance of pediatric patients with treatment involving antibiotic suspensions: a pilot study. *Clin Ther*. 1999; **21**: 1193–201.

Piglansky L, Leibovitz E, Raiz S, *et al*. Bacteriologic and clinical efficacy of high dose amoxicillin for therapy of acute otitis media in children. *Pediatr Infect Dis J*. 2003; **22**: 405–13.

Scottish Intercollegiate Guidelines Network (SIGN). *Community Management of Lower Respiratory Tract Infection in Adults*. Edinburgh: Scottish Intercollegiate Guidelines Network; 2002. Annex 1. www.sign.ac.uk/guidelines/published/support/guideline59/annex1.html (accessed 28 November 2011).

[5.1.1.3] Co-amoxiclav

Class:	β-lactamase-resistant broad-spectrum bactericidal antibacterial; a combination of amoxicillin and clavulanic acid
Tablet:	250/125 mg (= 375) or 500/125 mg (= 625)
Liquid:	400/57 mg in 5 mL
Dose:	adults: 375 mg 3 times a day
	increased to 625 mg in severe infections
	children **using 400/57 mg suspension** (be careful to specify the strength of the suspension as there are several types)
	7–12 years: 5 mL twice a day
	2–6 years: 2.5 mL twice a day
	2 months–2 years: 0.15 mL/kg twice a day
	paediatric doses should be doubled in severe infection
Pack:	21 tablets; 35, 70 mL liquid
$t_{1/2}$:	1 h (amoxicillin)
Side-effects:	nausea, diarrhoea, rashes, hepatitis, cholestatic jaundice: 1 in 6000 risk of liver damage (greater risk in men over 65 years of age, and with courses lasting over 2 weeks, but rare in children); also *see* phenoxymethylpenicillin, page 189
Interactions:	warfarin effect may be altered, **no** reduction in efficacy of oral contraceptives
Cautions:	penicillin allergy, liver or renal impairment: reduce dose for adults to twice daily if
	eGFR 10–30 and to once daily if
	eGFR < 10; for children with eGFR
	< 30 use an alternative antibiotic
Selection:	clavulanic acid is itself a β-lactam and can distract β-lactamase away from penicillins by acting as a decoy inhibitor, swamping the enzyme with false targets. Co-amoxiclav is useful when the broad spectrum of amoxicillin is required, but β-lactamase producing organisms, such as *S. aureus*, *H. influenzae*, *M. catarrhalis*, *E. coli* or *Bacteroides*, may be involved. It is the first choice for infected animal and human bites. If the infection is unlikely to involve bacteria producing β-lactamase, use plain amoxicillin instead because it is safer and cheaper

References

Andrade RJ, Tulkens PM. Hepatic safety of antibiotics used in primary care. *J Antimicrob Chemother*. 2011; **66**: 1431–46.

Garcia Rodriguez LA, Stricker BH, Zimmerman HJ. Risk of acute liver injury associated with the combination of amoxicillin and clavulanic acid. *Arch Intern Med*. 1996; **156**: 1327–33.

Medicines and Healthcare Products Regulatory Agency. *Curr Probl Pharmacovigilance*. 1993; **19**: 1–4.

[5.1.2] Cefalexin

Class:	cephalosporin β-lactamase-resistant broad-spectrum bactericidal antibacterial
Tablets or capsules:	250, 500 mg
Liquid:	125 mg/5 mL, 250 mg/5 mL
Dose:	adults: 250 mg 4 times a day, *or* 500 mg 2–3 times a day, increased in severe infection
	children 12–18 years: 500 mg 2–3 times a day, increased in severe infection
	5–12 years: 250 mg 3 times a day
	1–5 years: 125 mg 3 times a day
	1 month–1 year: 12.5 mg/kg twice a day, doubled in severe infection
Pack:	28 × 250 mg, 21 × 500 mg tablets or capsules; 100 mL liquid
$t_{1/2}$:	1 h
Side-effects:	rare, fever and joint pains; diarrhoea and rarely antibiotic-associated colitis, especially with high doses; or, with courses longer than 2 weeks, reduced white cells or platelets, liver or kidney damage which should recover once the drug is stopped
Interactions:	warfarin effect may be altered, **no** reduction in efficacy of oral contraceptives
Cautions:	immediate hypersensitivity to penicillin (use an alternative), renal impairment, porphyria. The efficacy of this antibiotic can be impaired by storage at high room temperatures
Selection:	cephalosporins are similar to β-lactamase-resistant penicillins in their action and their clinical use. Cefalexin is useful in treating urinary tract infections in pregnancy where the sensitivity of the infecting organism is not yet known and trimethoprim is not licensed for use. The frequently cited figure of 10% cross-reactivity between penicillin and cephalosporins is an overestimate (early cephalosporins were contaminated with penicillin moulds). The true figure is more like 0.5%. There may be a higher rate of cross-reactivity with completely unrelated antibiotics. Cephalosporins are broad-spectrum antibiotics that affect the normal gut flora and thereby increase the risk of antibiotic-associated diarrhoea. Where a good alternative exists, current advice from local microbiologists and public health consultants is to avoid cephalosporin. A link between primary care prescribing of oral cefalexin, often for only 3 days, in otherwise healthy adults and an increased incidence of *Clostridium difficile* is lacking. Cefalexin is currently one of the options recommended for treating lower urinary tract infection in pregnancy by Prodigy and *BNF*. In fact, there is good evidence that there is a greater increase in risk of *C. difficile* infection after quinolones (e.g ciprofloxacin), co-amoxiclav and later-generation cephalosporins, such as cefotaxime, rather than first-generation cephalosporins such as cefalexin

References

Crichton B. Keep in a cool place: exposure of medicines to high temperatures in general practice during a British heatwave. *J Roy Soc Med*. 2004; **97**(7): 328–9.

Pegler S, Healy B. In patients allergic to penicillin, consider second and third generation cephalosporins for life threatening infections. *BMJ*. 2007; **335**: 991.

Minson Q, Mok S. Relationship between antibiotic exposure and subsequent *Clostridium difficile*-associated diarrhoea. *Hosp Pharm*. 2007; **42**: 430–4.

[5.1.3] Doxycycline

Class:	tetracycline broad-spectrum bacteriostatic antibacterial
Capsules or dispersible tablets:	100 mg
Dose:	adults 200 mg on first day, then 100 mg daily. Capsules should be swallowed whole with plenty of fluid during meals, while sitting or standing, and at least 1 h before retiring to bed
Pack:	8
$t_{1/2}$:	16 (12–24) h (probably decreased by alcohol)
Side-effects:	photosensitivity (minimise exposure to strong sunlight or sunlamps) nausea, vomiting, dysphagia and oesophageal irritation (hence the instruction about how to take the medication); diarrhoea and rarely antibiotic-associated colitis; very rarely headache and visual disturbances which may indicate 'benign' intracranial hypertension, also rarely reported cases of hypoglycaemia in non-diabetic people
Interactions:	antacids (also quinapril which contains magnesium carbonate), iron, zinc, oral bismuth chelate (Pepto-Bismol® or De-Nol®), warfarin, antiepileptics, barbiturates, alcohol, rifampicin, **no** reduction in efficacy of oral contraceptives; avoid prescribing with ciclosporin or retinoids; avoid prescribing this bacteriostatic drug with a bactericidal antibiotic such as a penicillin, because the two mechanisms of action interfere with each other
Cautions:	**avoid prescribing in pregnancy**, breastfeeding, hepatic impairment, systemic lupus erythematosus (SLE), porphyria. **Not for children under 12 years of age**
Selection:	Doxycycline is well absorbed from the gut and not affected by food, or calcium-rich food which does affect other tetracyclines. It is eliminated via the bile and the faeces as well as in the urine, so there is no need to adjust the dose in mild or moderate renal impairment

References

Digre KB. Not so benign intracranial hypertension. *BMJ.* 2003; **326**(7390): 613–14.

Lochhead J, Elston JS. Doxycycline induced intracranial hypertension. *BMJ.* 2003; **326**(7390): 641–2.

Al-Mofarreh MA, Al Mofleh IA. Esophageal ulceration complicating doxycycline therapy. *World J Gastroenterol.* 2003; **9**(3): 609–11.

[5.1.5] Erythromycin – but generally use Clarithromycin (see notes under 'Selection')

Class:	macrolide bacteriostatic antibiotic
Enteric-coated tablets and capsules:	250, 500 mg
Liquid:	125 mg/5 mL, 250 mg/5 mL
Dose:	all 4 times a day, may be doubled for severe infections adults and children 8 years or older: 250 mg (if prescribing e/c tablets or capsules) children (liquid): 2–8 years, 250 mg 1 month–2 years: 125 mg
Pack:	28 tablets or capsules; 100, 140 mL liquid
$t_{1/2}$:	2 h
Side-effects:	nausea, vomiting, abdominal discomfort, diarrhoea (mainly after large doses), antibiotic-associated colitis; allergic reactions; reversible hearing loss also reported after large doses; if given for more than 14 days may occasionally cause cholestatic jaundice
Interactions:	amiodarone, **amlodipine (risk of hypotension)** atorvastatin, bromocriptine, buspirone, cabergoline, carbamazepine, cilostazol, **cimetidine**, clozapine, ciclosporin, digoxin, disopyramide, eletriptan, ergotamine, **felodipine, lercanidipine**, loratadine, mizolastine, midazolam, methysergide, **pimozide**, reboxetine, sertindole, sildenafil, **simvastatin**, sirolimus, tacrolimus, tadalafil, **theophylline**, vardenafil, **verapamil, warfarin**, zopiclone. There is no reduction in efficacy of oral contraceptives. Erythromycin and (to a lesser extent) clarithromycin interact with drugs which affect the enzyme CYP450 3A4 (see http://medicine.iupui.edu/clinpharm/ddis/table.aspx). If a macrolide antibiotic is needed in these patients, then azithromycin is the best choice
Cautions:	hepatic and severe renal impairment; avoid in porphyria
Selection:	this entry for erythromycin is retained in the formulary because the antibiotic is still in widespread use, but consider prescribing an alternative macrolide, clarithromycin or possibly azithromycin. One particular indication for this antibiotic is mastitis in a lactating woman who is allergic to penicillin because erythromycin has established safety in lactation. There have been a few reports of increased risk of pyloric stenosis but without sufficiently strong evidence to change prescribing. Clarithromycin is also safe in breast-feeding, but the manufacturers warn only to use if the benefit outweighs the potential risk, and caution is advised in the patient information leaflet, which can worry patients unnecessarily. For general use erythromcyin presents several problems. Gastrointestinal side-effects are common and there are multiple drug interactions. The only liquid form available is erythromycin ethyl succinate. Whereas the tablets and capsules are enteric-coated to protect the drug against destruction by gastric acid, the liquid form cannot be

enteric-coated, so doses for children are set to take into account this difference. The *BNF* and *BNFC* assume children under 8 years of age will be prescribed liquid. There are a number of preparations for adults without any evidence of one being superior to another, but there is a wide range in the prices. Generic enteric-coated tablets are the cheapest, but there will be a delay in onset of action until the tablet passes from the stomach into the small bowel. Capsules containing enteric-coated granules will have a faster onset, but are more expensive. Erythromycin binds to ribosomes within bacteria and interferes with protein synthesis. As Gram-positive organisms (e.g. streptococci, staphylococci) absorb the drug more readily, they are more susceptible to its action than Gram-negative ones. The spectrum of activity is similar to penicillin with additional activity against *Chlamydia* and unusual organisms such as *Mycoplasma* and *Legionella*, so it has often been suggested as a substitute when the patient is allergic to penicillin. This role is better served by clarithromycin as it avoids many of the problems associated with erythromycin. There is little difference in the cost of the generic drugs, but some formulations of erythromycin are considerably more expensive

References

[No authors listed]. Giving erythromycin by mouth. *Drug Ther Bull*. 1995; **33**(10): 77–9.

Langley JM, Halperin SA, Boucher FD, *et al*. Azithromycin is as effective as and better tolerated than erythromycin estolate for the treatment of pertussis. *Pediatrics*. 2004; **114**: e96–101.

Classen DC, Burke JP, Pestotnik SL, *et al*. Clinical and financial impact of intravenous erythromycin therapy in hospitalized patients. *Ann Pharmacother*. 1999; **33**: 669–73.

Carter BL, Woodhead JC, Cole KJ, *et al*. Gastrointestinal side-effects with erythromycin preparations. *Drug Intell Clin Pharm*. 1987; **21**: 734–8.

Wright AJ, Gomes T, Mamdani MM. The risk of hypotension following co-prescription of macrolide antibiotics and calcium-channel blockers. *CMAJ*. 2011; **183**(3): 303–7.

[5.1.5] Azithromycin

Class:	macrolide bacteriostatic antibacterial
Tablets:	250, 500 mg
Capsules:	250 mg
Liquid:	200 mg/5 mL
Dose:	**for general indications** all once a day for 3 days adults and children over 45 kg: 500 mg children 36–45 kg: 400 mg 26–35 kg: 300 mg 15–25 kg: 200 mg *or* over 6 months of age: 10 mg/kg once daily up to a maximum of 500 mg/day **for uncomplicated genital chlamydial infection and non-gonococcal urethritis** adults and children over 12 years: 1 g single dose
Pack:	4 × 250 mg, 6 × 250 mg, 3 × 500 mg tablets; 15, 30 mL liquid
$t_{1/2}$:	3 days
Side-effects:	less frequent than with erythromycin. Common side-effects are gut disturbances as with erythromycin, also anorexia, constipation. Most others are rare: pancreatitis, hepatitis, syncope, dizziness, headache, drowsiness, agitation, sensory disturbances, convulsions, blood abnormalities, kidney failure, joint aches, photosensitivity; rarely taste disturbances, tongue discolouration
Interactions:	azithromycin, unlike erythromycin and clarithromycin, does not inhibit liver enzymes, so interactions are much less of a problem. Antacids (avoid taking within 2 h of each other), ciclosporin, digoxin, ergotamine, theophylline, warfarin. There is no reduction in efficacy of oral contraceptives
Cautions:	avoid in liver disease. Inadequate evidence of safety in pregnancy and breastfeeding
Selection:	this macrolide is an alternative to others when interaction with other medication, such as statins or calcium channel blockers, needs to be avoided. It may also be useful for people who need help to take their medication, or those who strongly dislike taking medication. Its long half-life means that it can be given in a once-a-day dose, with a single dose for uncomplicated genital chlamydial infection, and the full course for general indications is just 3 days. It is more expensive than erythromycin or clarithromycin, but the time to recovery from acute tracheobronchitis is shorter. For female chlamydial infections, the improved compliance and lower risk of adverse reactions of azithromycin over doxycycline make it first choice. Erythromycin and (to a lesser extent) clarithromycin interact with drugs which affect the enzyme CYP450 3A4 (see http://medicine.iupui.edu/clinpharm/ddis/table.aspx). If a macrolide antibiotic is needed in these patients, then azithromycin is the best choice

References

Magid D, Douglas J, Schwartz S. Doxycycline compared with azithromycin for treating women with genital *Chlamydia trachomatis* infections: an incremental cost-effectiveness analysis. *Ann Int Med*. 1996; **124**: 389–99.

Sternon J, Leclerq P, Knepper C, *et al*. Azithromycin compared with clarithromycin in the treatment of patients with acute purulent tracheobronchitis: a cost of illness study. *J Int Med Res*. 1995; **23**: 413–22.

Langley JM, Halperin SA, Boucher FD, *et al*. Azithromycin is as effective as and better tolerated than erythromycin estolate for the treatment of pertussis. *Pediatrics*. 2004; **114**: e96–101.

[5.1.5] Clarithromycin

Class:	macrolide bacteriostatic antibacterial
Tablets:	250, 500 mg
Liquid:	125 mg/5 mL, 250 mg/5 mL
Dose:	all twice a day
	adults and children over 12 years: 250–500 mg
	children: *see* Table 12.1
Pack:	14 tablets; 70, 100 mL of 125 mg/5 mL; 70 mL of 250 mg/5 mL
$t_{\frac{1}{2}}$:	3 h after 250 mg; 9 h after 1200 mg
Side-effects:	less frequent than with erythromycin. Headache, taste disturbances, stomatitis, glossitis, hepatitis, phlebitis
Interactions:	**amlodipine (risk of hypotension)**, artemether/lumefantrine, atorvastatin, bromocriptine, cabergoline, carbamazepine, cimetidine, clozapine, ciclosporin, digoxin, disopyramide, eletriptan, ergotamine, felodipine, lercanidipine, itraconazole, methysergide, mizolastine, omeprazole, phenytoin, pimozide, reboxetine, repaglinide, rifabutin, sertindole, **simvastatin**, sirolimus, tacrolimus, tadalafil, terfenadine, theophylline, tolterodine, verapamil, **warfarin**, zopiclone. There is no reduction in efficacy of oral contraceptives. Erythromycin and (to a lesser extent) clarithromycin interact with drugs which affect the enzyme CYP450 3A4 (see http://medicine.iupui.edu/clinpharm/ddis/table.aspx). If a macrolide antibiotic is needed in these patients, then azithromycin is the best choice
Cautions:	hepatic and renal impairment. Avoid in porphyria
Selection:	clarithromycin is an erythromycin derivative with slightly greater activity than the parent compound and less risk of gastrointestinal side-effects. It is useful for people allergic to penicillin. It is better tolerated than erythromycin, the dosing is usually just twice daily, and without the need for enteric coating it will be absorbed more rapidly and reliably. Tissue concentrations are higher than with erythromycin. These are some of the reasons that it is recommended as the macrolide of choice in the British Thoracic Society guideline on treating community-acquired pneumonia

References

British Thoracic Society. Guidelines for the management of community acquired pneumonia in adults: update 2009. *Thorax*. 2009; **64**(Suppl. III): iii1–55.

Periti P, Mazzei T, Mini E, *et al*. Adverse effects of macrolide antibacterials. *Drug Saf*. 1993; **9**: 346–64.

Wright AJ, Gomes T, Mamdani MM. The risk of hypotension following co-prescription of macrolide antibiotics and calcium-channel blockers. *CMAJ*. 2011; **183**(3): 303–7.

TABLE 12.1 Children's doses of clarithromycin, all twice daily

Weight (kg)	Age (years)	Dose (mg)	Volume (mL) of 125 mg/5 mL	Volume (mL) of 250 mg/5 mL
30–40	10–12	250	10	5
20–29	6–9	187.5	7.5	–
12–19	2–5	125	5	–
8–11	1–2	62.5	2.5	–
under 8	under 1	7.5 mg/kg	0.3 mL/kg	–

[5.1.8] Trimethoprim

Class:	enzyme-inhibiting bacteriostatic antibacterial
Tablets:	100 mg, 200 mg
Liquid:	50 mg/5 mL
Dose:	all twice a day
	adults and children over 12 years: 200 mg
	children: 1 month–12 years 4 mg/kg (maximum 200 mg) (*see* Table 12.2)
Pack:	14 × 200 mg, 28 × 100 mg tablets (usually 6 for simple cystitis); 100 mL liquid
$t_{1/2}$:	10 h
Side-effects:	blood and generalised skin disorders, especially in the elderly or with long-term treatment; gastrointestinal disturbances including nausea and vomiting, allergic reactions, raised blood potassium
Interactions:	antimalarial drugs containing pyrimethamine (Fansidar® and Maloprim®), azathioprine, ciclosporin, mercaptopurine, **methotrexate**, phenytoin, warfarin. There is no reduction in efficacy of oral contraceptives
Cautions:	breastfeeding, renal impairment, avoid in pregnancy, porphyria, blood disorders. Use half normal dose after 3 days if eGFR 15–30 mL/min/1.73 m^2; use half normal dose if eGFR < 15 mL/min/1.73 m^2 (monitor plasma-trimethoprim concentration if eGFR < 10 mL/min/1.73 m^2)
Selection:	trimethoprim inhibits an enzyme (dihydrofolate reductase) that is essential for the metabolism of folic acid. It capitalises on the marked sensitivity of the bacterial enzyme relative to the human one. It should not be used in pregnancy because there is evidence of fetal abnormalities from animal studies, although many women have taken it before knowing they were pregnant and had no ill effects. Trimethoprim remains useful for treating uncomplicated urinary tract infections, but is inadequate for more serious ones, such as pyelonephritis. Although resistance is a problem (up to 30% in our locality), it may not be as great as it seems. Trimethoprim is more concentrated in urine than when it is used to test sensitivity in vitro, so a greater proportion of people treated empirically will be cured than predicted. It remains the first-line antibiotic to treat uncomplicated urinary tract infection in children. Its main advantages are that its narrow spectrum reduces the risk of antibiotic side-effects and it is so cheap as to be virtually free

References

Baerheim A. Empirical treatment of uncomplicated cystitis. *BMJ*. 2001; **323**: 1197–8.

Lawrenson RA, Logie JW. Antibiotic failure in the treatment of urinary tract infections in young women. *J Antimicrob Chem*. 2001; **48**: 895–901.

Lutters M, Vogt-Ferrier NB. Antibiotic duration for treating uncomplicated, symptomatic lower urinary tract infections in elderly women. *Cochrane Database Syst Rev*. 2002; **3**: CD001535.

Michael M, Hodson EM, Craig JC, *et al*. Short versus standard duration oral antibiotic therapy for acute urinary tract infection in children. *Cochrane Database Syst Rev*. 2003; **1**: CD003966. The Drug Safety. *Trimethoprim*. Available at: http://thedrugsafety.com/trimethoprim (accessed 11 August 2011).

TABLE 12.2 Example trimethoprim doses for children, all twice daily

Weight (kg)	Age (years)	Dose (mg)	Volume of 50 mg/5 mL
39	12	156	16
35	11	140	14
32	10	128	13
29	9	116	12
26	8	104	10
23	7	92	9
20	6	80	8
18	5	72	7
16	4	64	6
14	3	56	6
12	2	48	5
9	1	36	4
Under 9	1 month – 1 year	4 mg/kg	

[5.1.11] Metronidazole

Class:	azole bacteriostatic anti-anaerobic
Tablets:	200, 400 mg
Dose:	dental infections: 200 mg 3 times a day for 7 days
	bacterial vaginosis: 400 mg twice a day for 5 to 7 days or 2 g as a single dose (though a 1995 meta-analysis suggested that relapse rates were higher with a single dose). Different dosage regimens are used for other infections
Pack:	21
$t_{1/2}$:	8 h
Side-effects:	nausea (metallic taste in mouth), vomiting and gastrointestinal disturbances, rashes; rarely drowsiness, headache, dizziness, ataxia, hepatitis, blood disorders, aching, darkening of urine
Interactions:	alcohol (interaction may cause facial flushing, throbbing headache, palpitations, nausea and vomiting), warfarin, cimetidine, phenytoin, lithium. There is no reduction in efficacy of oral contraceptives
Cautions:	alcoholism, liver disease
Selection:	metronidazole is the first-line antibiotic used in the UK against anaerobic infections. In the context of treating minor illness, dental infections are quite commonly presented to health professionals other than dentists, and most acute cases of toothache involve infection, which can be appropriately treated with amoxicillin and/or metronidazole. Always advise the patient to consult a dentist, as without dental surgery the problem is likely to return after finishing the course of antibiotic

References

Joesoef MR, Schmid GP. Bacterial vaginosis: review of treatment options and potential clinical indications for therapy. *Clin Infect Dis.* 1995; **20**(Suppl. 1): S72–9.

Palmer NA, Pealing R, Ireland RS, *et al.* A study of therapeutic antibiotic prescribing in National Health Service general dental practice in England. *Br Dent J.* 2000; **188**(10): 554–8.

[5.1.13] Nitrofurantoin m/r

Class:	multiple-action bactericidal antibacterial
Modified release capsules:	100 mg
Dose:	100 mg twice a day for 3 days
Pack:	14 (but usual prescription is 6)
$t_{1/2}$:	20–30 min, but use of the modified-release version prolongs the action considerably
Side-effects:	urine may be coloured yellow or brown, anorexia, nausea and vomiting (modified release version less so), diarrhoea, acute and chronic pulmonary reactions, peripheral neuropathy; also reported rash, pruritus, hepatitis, pancreatitis, arthralgia, blood disorders and transient alopecia
Interactions:	magnesium trisilicate, probenecid, sulfinpyrazone. Patients should not take alkalinising agents such as Cymalon® with nitrofurantoin, as they reduce its effectiveness
Cautions:	renal failure (avoid if eGFR < 60; risk of peripheral neuropathy and ineffective because of inadequate urine concentrations), pregnancy at term, breastfeeding, glucose-6-phosphate dehydrogenase (G6PD) deficiency or porphyria; caution in anaemia, diabetes mellitus, electrolyte imbalance, vitamin B and folate deficiency, hepatic impairment, pulmonary disease, susceptibility to peripheral neuropathy. There is no reduction in efficacy of oral contraceptives
Selection:	only about 10% of bacteria responsible for UTI in general practice are resistant to nitrofurantoin. The antibacterial action of nitrofurantoin is unusual and not yet fully elucidated. Nitrofurantoin is converted to an active metabolite that interferes with many essential components of bacterial chemistry. Perhaps this multiple action accounts for the stable level of bacterial resistance, which has not increased appreciably since the antibacterial was first launched in 1953. As it is concentrated in the urine, it is highly effective against lower urinary tract infections, but the plasma levels are not sufficient to treat invasive infections such as pyelonephritis. It is as effective as broader-spectrum antibiotics without their significant risk of antibiotic-associated diarrhoea. It can be used in pregnancy but not at term because of a risk of neonatal haemolysis

References

Baerheim A. Empirical treatment of uncomplicated cystitis. *BMJ*. 2001; **323**: 1197–8.

Goettsch WG, Janknegt R, Hering RMC. Increased treatment failure after 3-days' courses of nitrofurantoin and trimethoprim for urinary tract infections in women: a population-based retrospective cohort study using the PHARMO database. *Br J Clin Pharmacol*. 2004; **58**: 184–9.

Gupta K, Hooton TM, Roberts PL, *et al*. Short-course nitrofurantoin for the treatment of acute uncomplicated cystitis in women. *Arch Intern Med*. 2007; **167**: 2207–12.

Spencer RC, Moseley DJ, Greensmith MJ. Nitrofurantoin modified release versus trimethoprim or co-trimoxazole in the treatment of uncomplicated urinary tract infection in general practice. *J Antimicrob Chemother*. 1994; **33**(Suppl. A): 121–9.

UK Teratology Service. *Use of Nitrofurantoin in Pregnancy*. 2010. Available at: www.toxbase.org/upload/Pregnancy pdfs/Nitrofurantoin 2010.pdf (accessed 12 September 2011).

Van Pinxteren B, Van Vliet SM, Wiersma TJ, *et al*. Summary of the practice guideline 'Urinary-tract infections' (second revision) from the Dutch College of General Practitioners. *Ned Tijdschr Geneeskd*. 2006; **150**: 718–22.

Zalmanovici Trestioreanu A, Green H, Paul M, *et al*. Antimicrobial agents for treating uncomplicated urinary tract infection in women. *Cochrane Database Syst Rev*. 2010, **10**: CD007182.

[5.2.1] Fluconazole (OTC)

Class:	triazole antifungal
Capsules:	50, 150 mg
Dose:	**for vaginal candidiasis**
	uncomplicated: 150 mg single dose
	for severe symptoms: 150 mg repeated after 3 days
	after alternative treatment failure: 100 mg/day for 7 days
	in poorly controlled diabetes or immunosuppression: 100 mg/day for 7 days
Pack:	1 × 150 mg, 7 × 50 mg
$t_{1/2}$:	30 h
Side-effects:	occasionally nausea, abdominal discomfort, diarrhoea, flatulence; rarely headache, hepatic disorders, skin reactions, seizures, reduced white cells or platelets, allergic reactions
Interactions:	avoid with eletroptan, pimozide, sertindole, sirolimus, tacrolimus. There are many interactions between triazole antifungal and other drugs, but most, with the exception of those listed, may be irrelevant to the use of a single dose of the antifungal
Cautions:	avoid in pregnancy and breastfeeding
Selection:	fluconazole is available OTC to people aged 16–60 years for the treatment of vaginal thrush and associated candidal balanitis as a single-dose pack of 150 mg. Some women find it more acceptable than using a clotrimazole pessary, but it is no more effective

References

Mendling W, Krauss C, Fladung B. A clinical multicenter study comparing efficacy and tolerability of topical combination therapy with clotrimazole (Canesten, two formats) with oral single dose fluconazole (Diflucan) in vulvovaginal mycoses. *Mycoses*. 2004; **47**: 136–42.

Nurbhai M, Grimshaw J, Watson M, *et al*. Oral versus intra-vaginal imidazole and triazole antifungal treatment of uncomplicated vulvovaginal candidiasis (thrush). *Cochrane Database Syst Rev*. 2007; **4**: CD002845.

[5.3.2.1] Aciclovir

Class:	antiviral
Tablets:	200, 400, 800 mg
Dispersible Tablets:	200, 400, 800 mg

Dose: **to treat varicella (chickenpox) or herpes zoster (shingles)**

adults and children over 12 years: 800 mg 5 times a day for 7 days (extend to 10 days if immunosuppressed, or nose or eye affected by shingles)
children 6–12 years: 800 mg 4 times a day for 5 days
2–6 years: 400 mg 4 times a day for 5 days
1 month–2 years: 200 mg 4 times a day for 5 days

Pack: 25×200 mg; 56×400 mg; 35×800 mg

$t_{\frac{1}{2}}$:   2–3 h

Side-effects: nausea, vomiting, abdominal pain, diarrhoea, headache, fatigue, fever, rash, urticaria, pruritus, photosensitivity; very rarely hepatitis, jaundice, dyspnoea, neurological reactions, acute renal failure, anaemia, thrombocytopenia and leucopenia

Interactions: minor interactions with ciclosporin, mycophenolate, probenecid, tacrolimus, theophylline

Cautions: renal impairment (dose interval may need to be increased if eGFR < 25), maintain adequate hydration, especially with higher doses; older people are more at risk of neurological reactions

Selection: aciclovir is active against herpes virus. The manufacturer advises caution in pregnancy and breastfeeding, but aciclovir is not known to be harmful. See the guideline referenced below for details on how to manage varicella in pregnancy. Dispersible tablets are suitable for children, but can also be prescribed for adults who prefer them; they are similar in price to the non-dispersible form

References

Breuer J, Fifer H. Chickenpox. *Clin Evid (Online)*. 2011; 201.

Klassen TP, Hartling L. Acyclovir for treating varicella in otherwise healthy children and adolescents. *Cochrane Database Syst Rev*. 2005; 4: CD002980.

Royal College of Obstetricians and Gynaecologists. *Chickenpox in Pregnancy*. 2007. Available at: www.rcog.org.uk/files/rcog-corp/uploaded-files/GT13ChickenpoxinPregnancy2007.pdf (accessed 13 August 2011).

[5.5.1] Mebendazole (OTC tablets only)

Class:	antihelmintic
Tablets (chewable):	100 mg
Liquid:	100 mg/5 mL
Dose:	**for threadworms**
	adults and children aged 2 years and older: 100 mg single dose (if reinfection occurs, a second dose may be needed after 2 weeks)
Pack:	6 tablets; 30 mL liquid
$t_{1/2}$:	1 h
Side-effects:	very rarely abdominal pain, diarrhoea, convulsions in infants, headache, dizziness, allergic reactions
Interactions:	cimetidine
Cautions:	avoid in pregnancy (toxicity in rats), no information about safety in breastfeeding
Selection:	this is the first-line treatment for treating threadworm infestations in anyone aged 2 years or over. It is not suitable for use in pregnancy because toxicity has been demonstrated in animal studies. As there is no suitable alternative treatment during early pregnancy, pregnant women have to rely on simple hygienic measures during the first trimester, but thereafter piperazine can be used. The *BNFC* includes the off-license use of mebendazole in children aged 6 months to 2 years, but the patient information leaflet in the Vermox® pack says that it is not suitable for children under 2 years, so prescribing it is likely to cause parental concern

References

Dawson M, Braithwaite PA, Roberts MS, *et al*. The pharmacokinetics and bioavailability of a tracer dose of [3H]-mebendazole in man. *Br J Clin Pharmacol*. 1985; **19**: 79–86.

Prodigy. *Clinical topic: Threadworm*. 2011. Available at: http://prodigy.clarity.co.uk/threadworm (accessed 11 August 2011).

[5.5.1] Piperazine + Senna (OTC)

Class:	antihelmintic
Oral powder:	for mixing into milk or water: piperazine phosphate 4 g, sennosides 15.3 mg per sachet
Dose:	**for threadworms**
	2 doses are given, two weeks apart
	adults: 1 sachet at bedtime
	children aged 2 years or older: use mebendazole
	1 year–1 year 11 months: 5 mL of sachet contents in the morning
	3 months–1 year: 2.5 mL of sachet contents in the morning
Pack:	2 sachets
$t_{\frac{1}{2}}$:	wide variation between individuals, but usually fully eliminated within 24 h
Side-effects:	nausea, vomiting, colic, diarrhoea, allergic reactions, seizures, incoordination, vertigo, blurred vision, drowsiness, confusion
Interactions:	none
Cautions:	avoid in liver impairment, first trimester of pregnancy (manufacturer's advice), severe renal impairment, or epilepsy; if breastfeeding, express and discard breast milk for 8 h after the dose
Selection:	this is the alternative treatment for threadworm infestations when mebendazole cannot be used

Reference

Leach FN. Management of threadworm infestation during pregnancy [review]. *Arch Dis Child*. 1990; **65**: 399–400.

Endocrine system

[6.3.2] Prednisolone

Class: corticosteroid

Tablets: 5 mg

Soluble tablets: 5 mg

Dose: **severe hay fever not responding to other treatments, or for short-term relief for important events**

adults and children over 12 years: 15–20 mg daily
children 6–12 years: 5–10 mg daily
the British Society for Allergy and Clinical Immunology (BSACI) guideline on allergic rhinitis suggests a dose for adults of 0.5 mg/kg given orally in the morning with food for 5–10 days, and this could be extended to children, but *Drug and Therapeutics Bulletin* recommends using the minimum effective dose up to a maximum dose of 20 mg daily. At the NMIC, we have found that the lower doses recommended above are usually adequate to control symptoms

acute exacerbation of asthma
adults and children over 12 years: 40–50 mg daily for at least 5 days until recovery
children 6–12 years: 30–40 mg daily for 3 days
2–5 years: 20 mg for 3 days
under 2 years: 10 mg for 3 days

acute exacerbation of COPD
adults: 30 mg daily for 14 days

croup
children: two doses 24 h apart of 1–2 mg/kg

Pack: 28 tablets, 30 soluble tablets

$t_{1/2}$: 2–3 h, but the effect lasts considerably longer

Side-effects: corticosteroids demonstrate many different types of side-effect: on starting treatment (psychiatric reactions, loss of diabetic control), on continuing treatment (osteoporosis, Cushingoid features, fragile skin), and on stopping (Addisonian crisis, mood changes). However, the durations of treatment for the indications above are short enough that treatment can be stopped abruptly at the end of the course. For a full list of possible side-effects, see the notes to section 6.3.2 of the *BNF*

Interactions: corticosteroids have such manifest effects that many interactions occur. These do not usually preclude the use of high-dose short-term treatments for the above indications. In summary, expect a deterioration in control of blood pressure, diabetes, anticoagulation, epilepsy; an increased risk of gastrointestinal bleeding from NSAIDs; hypokalaemia is more likely with concomitant theophyllines, salbutamol or diuretics like furosemide or bendroflumethiazide, and the effect of this exacerbates digoxin toxicity

Cautions: previous severe mental illness; dosage may need reducing in chronic liver or kidney disease. Patient should avoid contact with chickenpox while taking prednisolone unless they are known to be immune

Selection: prescribe standard 5 mg tablets, or if the patient needs a liquid form, soluble tablets. There is no advantage in using enteric-coated tablets as the tenuous link to peptic ulceration would be a systemic effect of the drug, not a local one on the gastric mucosa, and there is possible delayed or non-absorption from such a formulation. Injections offer no advantage over tablets unless the patient is vomiting or cannot swallow, and there is a disadvantage of possible allergic reactions to parenteral hydrocortisone

References

[No authors listed]. Any place for depot triamcinolone in hay fever? *Drug Ther Bull*. 1999; 37(3): 17–18.

British Thoracic Society, Scottish Intercollegiate Guidelines Network. *BTS/SIGN Asthma Guideline*. 2011. Available at: www.brit-thoracic.org.uk/guidelines/asthma-guidelines.aspx (accessed 11 August 2011).

National Institute for Health and Clinical Excellence. *Chronic Obstructive Pulmonary Disease (updated): NICE guideline 101*. London: NIHCE; 2010. www.nice.org.uk/guidance/CG101 (accessed 28 November 2011).

Scadding GK, Durham SR, Mirakianz R, *et al*. BSACI guidelines for the management of allergic and non-allergic rhinitis. *Clin Exp Allergy*. 2008; 38: 19–42.

[6.4.1.2] Norethisterone

Class:	progestogen
Tablets:	5 mg
Dose:	**to delay menstruation:** 5 mg 3 times a day, starting 3 days before expected menstrual period
Pack:	30
$t_{1/2}$:	8 (5–12) h
Side-effects:	fluid retention, weight gain, nausea, change in libido, breast discomfort, headache, dizziness, insomnia, drowsiness, depression, skin reactions including exacerbation of acne, jaundice, allergic reactions
Interactions:	ciclosporin, warfarin, antidiabetic drugs; drugs that accelerate the metabolism of progestogens and reduce the effectiveness of progestogen-only contraceptives could reduce the effectiveness of norethisterone used to delay a period
Cautions:	pregnancy, breastfeeding, arterial disease, susceptibility to thromboembolism, epilepsy, uncontrolled hypertension, cardiac failure, renal or liver impairment, migraine, depression, diabetes
Selection:	norethisterone is useful to delay an inconvenient period. Side-effects are quite common but usually mild, with breast tenderness and fluid retention. Bleeding occurs 2–3 days after stopping the norethisterone. Women taking a standard combined oral contraceptive pill do not need norethisterone for this purpose; they can simply continue without having a 7-day gap between packs. Norethisterone is a synthetic progestogen related to testosterone. Be aware that there has been some publicity that such progestogens may cause an increased risk of breast cancer, but there is no good evidence for this claim

Reference

Kuhl H. Scientific comment: norethisterone acetate (NETA) – a risky compound? *Geburtsh Frauenheilk*. 2000; **60**: 393–406.

Obstetrics and gynaecology

[7.2.2] Clotrimazole (OTC)

Class:	imidazole antifungal
External cream:	2%
Pessaries:	200, 500 mg
Intravaginal cream:	10%
Dose:	for vaginal candidiasis
	uncomplicated: 500 mg pessary or 5 g of 10% intravaginal cream inserted at night
	for severe symptoms: 500 mg pessary inserted at night, repeated after 3 days
	after alternative treatment failure: 200 mg pessary inserted at night for 6 nights
	in poorly controlled diabetes or immunosuppression: 200 mg pessary inserted at night for 6 nights
	pregnancy: 200 mg pessary each night for 7 nights
Pack:	20 g external cream; one 500 mg pessary with applicator; combination pack with 1 pessary and 10 g external cream; vaginal cream 5 g with applicator
Side-effects:	possible destructive effect on latex condoms and diaphragms (use alternative contraception for at least 5 days after dose), local irritation; rarely allergic reactions
Interactions:	none
Cautions:	occasionally development of sensitivity to one of the excipients may produce symptoms similar to the original infection
Selection:	the usual treatment for vaginal thrush is a single dose of a 500 mg pessary inserted at night. Some women may prefer to use the 10% vaginal cream. External infection can be treated with 2% cream, but this is not sufficient if, as is often the case, there is concurrent vaginal infection. Clotrimazole can be used in pregnancy

References

British Association for Sexual Health and HIV (BASHH). *National Guideline on the Management of Vulvovaginal Candidiasis*. 2007. Available at: www.bashh.org/documents/50/50.pdf (accessed 3 August 2011).

Nurbhai M, Grimshaw J, Watson M, *et al*. Oral versus intra-vaginal imidazole and triazole anti-fungal treatment of uncomplicated vulvovaginal candidiasis (thrush). *Cochrane Database Syst Rev*. 2007; **4**: CD002845.

Young G, Jewell D. Topical treatment for vaginal candidiasis (thrush) in pregnancy. *Cochrane Database Syst Rev*. 2001; **4**: CD000225.

[7.2.2] Metronidazole vaginal gel

Class:	azole bacteriostatic anti-anaerobic
Vaginal gel:	0.75%
Dose:	5 g application at night for 5 nights
Pack:	40 g with applicators
Side-effects:	local irritation, candidiasis, abnormal discharge, abdominal or pelvic discomfort, possibly decreased appetite, headache, dizziness, nausea
Interactions:	unlikely to affect systemic medications as little is absorbed
Cautions:	not for use during menstruation, hypersensitivity to metronidazole, concomitant candidiasis would need oral treatment, sexual intercourse not recommended during treatment period
Selection:	topical treatment for bacterial vaginosis is as effective as oral metronidazole. It is considered safe in pregnancy and breastfeeding. Only if there is a problem using metronidazole would the alternative of clindamycin be used. They are equally effective, but clindamycin is more expensive and more likely to generate resistant strains (for reference, see next entry for clindamycin)

Reference

Joesoef MR, Schmid GP, Hillier SL. Bacterial vaginosis: review of treatment options and potential clinical indications for therapy. *Clin Infect Dis.* 1999; **28**(Suppl. 1): S57–65.

[7.2.2] Clindamycin vaginal cream

Class:	lincosamide bacteriostatic antibiotic
Vaginal cream:	2%
Dose:	5 g application at night for 7 nights
Pack:	40 g with applicators
Side-effects:	local irritation, cervicitis, vaginitis, abdominal or pelvic discomfort, possibly rash, headache, dizziness, vertigo, heartburn, nausea, diarrhoea, constipation
Interactions:	unlikely to affect systemic medications as little is absorbed
Cautions:	damages latex condoms and diaphragms, hypersensitivity to clindamycin, manufacturer advises against use during menstruation or the first trimester of pregnancy, but considered safe in breastfeeding
Selection:	topical treatment for bacterial vaginosis is as effective as oral metronidazole. Only if there is a problem using metronidazole would the alternative of clindamycin be used. They are equally effective, but clindamycin is more expensive and more likely to generate resistant strains

References

Austin MN, Beigi RH, Meyn LA, *et al.* Microbiological response to treatment of bacterial vaginosis with topical clindamycin or metronidazole. *J Clin Microbiol.* 2005; **43**: 4492–7. doi: 10.1128/JCM.43.9.4492-4497.2005 Available at: http://jcm.asm.org/content/43/9/4492.full (accessed 29 November 2011).

Paavonen J, Mangioni C, Martin MA, *et al.* Vaginal clindamycin and oral metronidazole for bacterial vaginosis: a randomised trial. *Obstet Gynaecol.* 2005; **96**(2): 256–60 www.ncbi.nlm.nih.gov/pubmed/10908773 (accessed 29 November 2011).

[7.3.5] Levonorgestrel (OTC for a woman over 16 years)

Class:	post-coital contraceptive – progestogen
Tablets:	1.5 mg
Dose:	1.5 mg as soon as possible after unprotected sexual intercourse, and not later than 72 h after
Pack:	1 tablet
$t_{1/2}$:	10 (9–14.5) h
Side-effects:	nausea (affecting 14%–23% of patients; if vomiting occurs efficacy may be lost – if vomiting occurs within 2 h of intake, another tablet should be taken with domperidone), lower abdominal pain (18%), fatigue (17%), headache (17%), dizziness (11%), breast tenderness (11%), vomiting (6%). Glucose tolerance may worsen. The timing of menstrual bleeding may be temporarily disturbed, although most women have their next period on time. If it is more than 1 week overdue, a pregnancy test is needed. A barrier method will need to be used until the next period. Also advise the patient to report any lower abdominal pains, which might indicate an ectopic pregnancy
Interactions:	drugs that induce liver enzymes reduce the effectiveness of the contraception. The drugs suspected of doing this are: carbamazepine, griseofulvin, phenytoin, primodone, rifabutin, rifampicin, ritonavir, St John's Wort. If levonorgestrel is still considered the best option, the dose needs to be increased to 3 mg (unlicensed dose). There is also an interaction with ciclosporin, which could lead to toxic effects
Cautions:	check that there was no earlier unprotected intercourse during the same cycle that would be outside the time limit. Also check that a period is not overdue, which may be because the woman is already pregnant. Severe malabsorption, such as in severe Crohn's disease, could affect the absorption of the drug. Avoid in pregnancy, porphyria or severe liver disease. Caution if past history of salpingitis or ectopic pregnancy
Selection:	levonorgestrel in a single dose of 1.5 mg provides post-coital contraception when taken after unprotected sexual intercourse. The earlier it is taken the better, but the overall effectiveness if taken within 72 h of unprotected sex is 69%–85% of expected pregnancies are prevented. It is less effective for women with a high body mass index. Between 72–120 h, use ulipristal instead. The main alternative is an IUCD. The manufacturer's website provides a calculator to show the timeframe during which Levonelle One Step can be taken and where to obtain it within a locality. There is limited information on use by women under 16 years of age, but all available methods of emergency contraception should be offered to women attending for it, regardless of age, as the risk of an unwanted pregnancy outweighs that of the contraceptive

References

Faculty of Sexual & Reproductive Healthcare. *Contraceptive Choices for Young People: clinical guidance*. 2010. Available at: www.fsrh.org/pdfs/ceuGuidanceYoungPeople2010.pdf (accessed 14 August 2011).

Kozinszky Z, Bakken RT, Lieng M. Ectopic pregnancy after levonorgestrel emergency contraception. *Contraception*. 2011; **83**: 281–3.

Piaggio G, Kapp N, Von Hertzen H. Effect on pregnancy rates of the delay in the administration of levonorgestrel for emergency contraception: a combined analysis of four WHO trials. *Contraception*. 2011; **84**: 35–9.

Von Hertzen H, Piaggio G, Ding J, *et al*. Low dose mifepristone and two regimens of levonorgestrel for emergency contraception: a WHO multicentre randomised trial. *Lancet*. 2002; **360**: 1803–10.

Webb A, Shochet T, Bigrigg A, *et al*. Effect of hormonal emergency contraception on bleeding patterns. *Contraception*. 2004; **69**: 133–5.

www.levonelle.co.uk (accessed 28 November 2011).

[7.3.5] Ulipristal

Class:	post-coital contraceptive – progesterone receptor blocker (partial agonist)
Tablets:	30 mg
Dose:	30 mg as soon as possible after unprotected sexual intercourse, and usually not later than 120 h after
Pack:	1 tablet
$t_{\frac{1}{2}}$:	32 (26–39) h
Side-effects:	gastrointestinal disturbance (note: if vomiting occurs efficacy may be lost – if vomiting occurs within 3 h of intake, another tablet should be taken with domperidone), next menstrual period may be early or late by a few days, dizziness, mood changes, fatigue, headache, back pain, muscle spasm, occasionally tremor, hot flushes, uterine spasm, breast tenderness, dry mouth, blurred vision, pruritus, rash
Interactions:	St John's wort, proton pump inhibitors (e.g. omeprazole), ranitidine, antacids, antiepileptic drugs may result in decrease in efficacy
Cautions:	not for use in pregnancy, or coincident severe asthma not adequately controlled, recommend use of barrier method of contraception for rest of cycle as the action of hormonal contraceptive can be affected. Advise a lactating woman to express and discard breast milk for 36 h after a dose of ulipristal
Selection:	this new post-coital contraceptive is licensed for use up to 5 days after unprotected sexual intercourse – 2 days more than levonorgestrel. As there is less information about this contraceptive than levonorgestrel, and increased cost, levonorgestrel remains the first-line choice up to the 3-day limit. Beyond this, a copper intrauterine device is suitable up to 5 days after the earliest likely calculated ovulation, and ulipristal is an option between 3 and 5 days after unprotected sexual intercourse. The earlier it is taken the better, but the overall effectiveness if taken within 120 h of unprotected sex is that 85% of expected pregnancies are prevented. It is less effective for women with a high body mass index. There is limited information on use by women under 18 years of age, but all available methods of emergency contraception should be offered to women attending for it, regardless of age, as the risk of an unwanted pregnancy outweighs that of the contraceptive

References

Drug and Therapeutics Bulletin. Ulipristal: a new emergency contraceptive pill. *Drug Ther Bull*. 2010; 48: 86–8.

Faculty of Sexual & Reproductive Healthcare. *Contraceptive Choices for Young People: clinical guidance*. 2010. Available at: www.fsrh.org/pdfs/ceuGuidanceYoungPeople2010.pdf (accessed 14 August 2011).

Faculty of Sexual & Reproductive Healthcare. *New Product Review: ulipristal acetate (ellaOne®)*. 2009. Available at: www.fsrh.org/pdfs/ellaOneNewProductReview1009.pdf (accessed 14 August 2011).

Nutrition and blood

[9.1.1] Ferrous fumarate (OTC)

Best prescribed as Fersaday® (but first check your local pharmacy can supply it)

Class: iron

Capsules: 322 mg

Dose: adults only: 322 mg twice a day before food

Pack: 28

$t_{1/2}$: not applicable as iron is used and stored within the body rather than eliminated

Side-effects: **reduce dose if side-effects occur** – nausea, epigastric pain, constipation (particularly in the elderly) or diarrhoea

Interactions: reduced absorption of iron with magnesium trisilicate, tetracyclines, and zinc, trientine. Iron reduces absorption of tetracyclines (e.g. doxycycline), quinolone antibiotics (e.g. ciprofloxacin), **levothyroxine** (take iron and levothyroxine at least 2 h apart), L-dopa, entacapone, biphosphonates, penicillamine and zinc

Cautions: dangerous to children in overdose

Selection: this is only used for treating iron deficiency, which usually manifests as microcytic anaemia. A low haemoglobin level frequently occurs in pregnancy, due to dilution. If the mean cell volume is normal, iron deficiency is unlikely. Side-effects are related to the dose of iron rather than the formulation. Taking the iron with food reduces both the absorption and the chance of side-effects. There is no point in advocating a diet rich in vitamin C to help improve the absorption, because this only works by converting ferric iron in food to the more readily absorbed ferrous form. As ferrous fumarate is already in this form, adding vitamin C gives no advantage. Prescribing the Fersaday brand ensures a blister pack, which reduces the potentially fatal risk of iron poisoning in infants who manage to get hold of their parent's medication

References

Mahomed K. Iron and folate supplementation in pregnancy. *Cochrane Database Syst Rev.* 2006; **3**: CD001135.

Tenenbein M. Unit-dose packaging of iron supplements and reduction of iron poisoning in young children. *Arch Pediatr Adolesc Med.* 2005; **159**: 557–60.

[9.2.1.2] Dioralyte® (OTC)

Class: oral rehydration

Sachets: blackcurrant, citrus or natural; mix one sachet with 200 mL drinking water, use within 1 hour or keep in fridge for up to 24 h

Dose: according to fluid loss, but usually

adults: 200–400 mL after every loose motion

children 2–12 years: 200 mL after every loose motion

infants up to 2 years: 1–1.5 times usual feed volume

Pack: 6 or 20

Side-effects: potentially electrolyte imbalance could arise if the solution was incorrectly diluted

Interactions: none

Cautions: none

Selection: having experienced the distribution of a recipe by a health authority for a home-made oral rehydration fluid mixture only to see it rapidly withdrawn when it was discovered that the quantity of salt was incorrect, using manufactured sachets containing the correct amount is clearly a safer option. If professionals can get the mixture wrong, then so can parents. For those who are normally healthy in affluent countries with plentiful drinking water, oral rehydration with electrolyte-water mixtures is rarely necessary; what matters is maintaining adequate fluid intake and restarting feeding as soon as possible. Note that rehydration fluids used in Britain have less salt and more glucose than the World Health Organization formulation

References

Hahn S, Kim Y, Garner P. Reduced osmolarity oral rehydration solution for treating dehydration due to diarrhoea in children: systematic review. *BMJ*. 2001; **323**: 81–5.

Ho TF, Yip WCL, Duggan C, *et al.* Letters about oral rehydration solutions. *BMJ*. 2001; **323**: 1068.

Mecrow IK, Miller V. An open triple crossover study comparing water absorption from potable water, Lucozade, and Dioralyte using the stable isotope 18O. *J Pediatr Gastroenterol Nutr*. 1993; **16**: 316–20.

Musculoskeletal system

[10.1.1] Ibuprofen (OTC)

Class:	non-steroidal anti-inflammatory drug
Tablets:	200, 400, 600 mg
Liquid:	100 mg/5 mL
Dose:	all 3 times a day, increasing to 4 times only if necessary
	adults: 400–600 mg
	children 12–18 years: 300–400 mg
	10–12 years: 300 mg (15 mL)
	7–10 years: 200 mg (10 mL)
	4–7 years: 150 mg (7.5 mL)
	1–4 years: 100 mg (5 mL)
	3 months–1 year: 50 mg (2.5 mL)

approximately equivalent to 20 mg per kg body weight per day, not licensed for children under 3 months of age or weighing under 5 kg

Pack:	84 tablets (but only prescribe the amount required); 100, 150, 500 mL liquid
$t_{1/2}$:	2 h
Side-effects:	gastrointestinal discomfort – also nausea, diarrhoea, and occasionally bleeding and ulceration, hypersensitivity reactions – notably with bronchospasm, rashes and angio-oedema. Other rare side-effects include fluid retention, headache, dizziness, vertigo, changes in mood, hearing disturbances such as tinnitus, photosensitivity, haematuria, blood disorders, renal failure, alveolitis, hepatic damage, pancreatitis, eye changes and aseptic meningitis. High doses are associated with an increased risk of cardiovascular events
Interactions:	ibuprofen co-administered with **aspirin** can not only increase the risk of gastrointestinal haemorrhage but may also counteract the protective effect of aspirin against thrombosis. Other interactions with: antihypertensives and diuretics may have reduced effectiveness and increased risk of NSAID-induced renal toxicity, ciclosporin, **clopidogrel**, corticosteroids, digoxin, lithium, methotrexate, penicillamine, pentoxyifylline, phenytoin, quinolones (e.g. ciprofloxacin), SSRI antidepressants (such as fluoxetine), sulphonylureas (such as gliclazide), tacrolimus, **warfarin**
Cautions:	**avoid prescribing in the presence of:**

- gastrointestinal disease – especially a history of peptic ulcer, GI bleed or inflammatory bowel disease
- allergy to aspirin or other NSAID
- severe kidney disease (eGFR < 30)
- severe liver disease
- heart failure
- taking prophylactic aspirin or warfarin

- chickenpox or shingles – increased risk of serious secondary skin infection with NSAIDs
- pregnancy or trying to conceive

use with caution if:
- older patients – risk of gastrointestinal bleeding higher, especially in older men
- hypertension
- ischaemic heart disease
- recovering from surgery, fracture or injury
- systemic lupus erythematosus
- breastfeeding
- asthma: about 5% of adults find that aspirin causes or exacerbates wheezing. There is a concern that the same effect may occur with ibuprofen and other NSAIDs. There are a few case reports of such, but despite frequent mention in reviews there is little hard evidence. Furthermore, children have fewer problems with asthma when febrile illnesses are treated with ibuprofen instead of paracetamol. The exacerbation of asthma caused by ibuprofen in individuals who are not specifically allergic to it may turn out to be as much a myth as the misconception that ibuprofen was once claimed to be ineffective in women

Selection: of the group of standard NSAIDs, ibuprofen poses the least risk of gastrointestinal bleeding. Toxicity to the gut is mainly from the systemic effect of ibuprofen, not a local effect, so it makes little difference whether it is taken after food or not. There is no reason to recommend that young children are given paracetamol in addition to ibuprofen to control fever, and NICE advises against this combination. Consider co-prescribing a proton pump inhibitor (e.g. omeprazole) even for short courses in older people or anyone with a higher than average risk of peptic ulceration or bleeding. Cardiovascular risks with ibuprofen are associated with higher doses

References

[No authors listed]. Mythbuster: ibuprofen and women. *Bandolier*. 2004; **120**: 4.

[No authors listed]. Varicella, herpes zoster and nonsteroidal anti-inflammatory drugs: serious cutaneous complications [review]. *Prescribe Int*. 2010; **19**(106): 72–3.

Body R, Potier K. Non-steroidal anti-inflammatory drugs and exacerbations of asthma in children. *Emerg Med J*. 2004; **21**: 713.

Debley JS, Carter ER, Gibson RL, *et al*. The prevalence of ibuprofen-sensitive asthma in children: a randomized controlled bronchoprovocation challenge study. *J Pediatr*. 2006; **148**(5): 704–5; author reply 705–6.

Farkouh ME, Greenberg JD, Jeger RV, *et al*. Cardiovascular outcomes in high risk patients with osteoarthritis treated with ibuprofen, naproxen or lumiracoxib. *Ann Rheum Dis*. 2007; **66**: 764–70.

Hay AD, Costelloe C, Redmond NM, *et al.* Paracetamol plus ibuprofen for the treatment of fever in children (PITCH): randomised controlled trial. *BMJ.* 2008; **337**: a1302.

Khazaeinia T, Jamali F. Evaluation of gastrointestinal toxicity of ibuprofen using surrogate markers in rats: effect of formulation and route of administration. *Clin Exp Rheumatol.* 2000; **18**: 187–92.

Kwok CK, Feinstein AR. Rates of sensitivity reactions to aspirin: problems in interpreting the data. *Clin Pharmacol Ther.* 1986; **40**: 494–505.

MacDonald TM, Wei L. Effect of ibuprofen on cardioprotective effect of aspirin. *Lancet.* 2003; **361**: 57.

Mikaeloff Y, Kezouh A, Suissa S. Nonsteroidal anti-inflammatory drug use and the risk of severe skin and soft tissue complications in patients with varicella or zoster disease. *Br J Clin Pharmacol.* 2008; **65**: 203–9.

National Institute for Health and Clinical Excellence. *Feverish Illness in Children: assessment and the initial management in children younger than 5 years. NICE guideline 47.* London: NIHCE; 2007. www.nice.org.uk/guidance/CG47 (accessed 28 November 2011).

[10.1.1] Naproxen (OTC – 9 × 250 mg for dysmenorrhoea in women aged 15–50)

Class:	non-steroidal anti-inflammatory drug
Tablets:	250, 500 mg
Dose:	adults and children over 16 years: 500 mg initially, then 250 mg every 6–8 h
Pack:	28
$t_{1/2}$:	12–15 h
Side-effects:	gastrointestinal discomfort – also nausea, diarrhoea, and occasionally bleeding and ulceration, hypersensitivity reactions – notably with bronchospasm, rashes and angio-oedema. Other rare side-effects include fluid retention, headache, dizziness, vertigo, changes in mood, hearing disturbances such as tinnitus, haematuria, blood disorders, hyperkalaemia, renal failure, alveolitis, hepatic damage, pancreatitis, eye changes and aseptic meningitis
Interactions:	as for ibuprofen
Cautions:	as for ibuprofen
Selection:	naproxen is an alternative NSAID to ibuprofen, with higher potency, higher risk of gastrointestinal bleeding, but a relatively low risk of cardiac ischaemic events compared with other NSAIDs. It is not affected by gastric acid and therefore does not need to be given in an enteric-coated form, so is faster acting than diclofenac e/c. The comparatively long half-life means it can be taken twice daily. Consider co-prescribing a proton pump inhibitor (e.g. omeprazole) even for short courses in older people or anyone with a higher than average risk of peptic ulceration or bleeding

References

Hawkey CJ, Hawkey GM, Everitt S, *et al*. Increased risk of myocardial infarction as first manifestation of ischaemic heart disease and nonselective nonsteroidal anti-inflammatory drugs. *Br J Clin Pharmacol*. 2006; **61**: 730–7.

Lethaby A, Augood C, Duckitt K, *et al*. Nonsteroidal anti-inflammatory drugs for heavy menstrual bleeding. *Cochrane Database Syst Rev*. 2007; **4**: CD000400.

Pilotto A, Franceschi M, Leandro G, *et al*. The risk of upper gastrointestinal bleeding in elderly users of aspirin and other non-steroidal anti-inflammatory drugs: the role of gastroprotective drugs. *Aging Clin Exp Res*. 2003; **15**: 494–9.

Ray WA, Varas-Lorenzo C, Chung CP, *et al*. Cardiovascular risks of nonsteroidal antiinflammatory drugs in patients after hospitalization for serious coronary heart disease. *Circ Cardiovasc Qual Outcomes*. 2009; **2**: 155–63.

[10.3.2] Ketoprofen (topical) (OTC)

Class:	topical non-steroidal anti-inflammatory drug
Gel:	2.5%
Dose:	apply 2–4 times daily for 1 week
Pack:	30, 50, 100 g
$t_{1/2}$:	although the plasma half-life is 2 h, levels in the blood are very low with topical formulations
Side-effects:	**photosensitivity** – patients should be warned to wash hands thoroughly after application and avoid sun exposure, even if cloudy, to the area treated, during and for 2 weeks after stopping treatment; rarely, allergic reactions including asthma and rashes; dyspepsia, exacerbation of renal impairment
Interactions:	most unlikely with topical form
Cautions:	avoid if known hypersensitivity to aspirin or other NSAIDs; do not apply to areas of damaged skin; do not apply to mucous membranes, anal or genital areas, eyes or use with occlusive dressings
Selection:	topical NSAIDs can be detected at therapeutically effective concentration to a depth of 3 cm in soft tissue under the area of application and for at least 15 h after application. Concentrations of the drug local to the area of application are likely to be at least as high as if an oral dose had been taken, but there is hardly any penetration into large joints. Therefore, the percutaneous route is ideal for soft tissue inflammatory conditions but not suitable for relieving arthritic pain. Gel formulations provide better absorption than emulsions. There is evidence that ketoprofen is more effective than other topical NSAIDs and it is available generically at low cost

References

Bandolier. *Topically Applied Non-steroidal Anti-inflammatory Drugs in Acute Pain*. 1999. Available at: www.medicine.ox.ac.uk/bandolier/booth/painpag/Acutrev/Other/AP020.html (accessed 11 August 2011).

Dominkus M, Nicolakis M, Kotz R, *et al.* Comparison of tissue and plasma levels of ibuprofen after oral and topical administration. *Arzneimittel-Forsch.* 1996; **46**: 1138–43.

Mason L, Moore RA, Edwards JE, *et al.* Topical NSAIDs for acute pain: a meta-analysis. *BMC Fam Pract.* 2004; **5**: 10.

Treffel P, Gabard B. Ibuprofen epidermal levels after topical application in vitro: effect of formulation, application time, dose variation and occlusion. *Br J Dermatol.* 1993; **129**: 286–91.

Vaile JH, Davis P. Topical NSAIDs for musculoskeletal conditions. A review of the literature. *Drugs.* 1998; **56**: 783–99.

Eye

[11.3.1] Chloramphenicol (OTC drops for adults and children 2 years and over)

Class:	topical, primarily bacteriostatic, antibiotic
Drops:	0.5%
Ointment:	1%
Dose:	drops: apply hourly at first, reduce to 4-hourly as symptoms improve
	ointment: apply 4 times a day, or at night if used in conjunction with drops
Pack:	10 mL drops or 4 g ointment
$t_{1/2}$:	5 h – but not relevant to topical use because so little is absorbed
Side-effects:	transient stinging
Interactions:	none
Cautions:	past or close family history of blood disorder. In pregnancy, topical fusidic acid is preferred
Selection:	chloramphenicol has a broad spectrum of activity, but its systemic use is limited by rare but serious toxicity. Topical use is free from this hazard. The risk of serious blood disorders among people who have used topical chloramphenicol is no higher than the background rate, but the reassurance gained from this does not necessarily apply to patients who have a past or close family history of such disorders, who could be more susceptible. The patient information leaflet warns of this

References

Laporte JR, Vidal X, Ballarin E, *et al*. Possible association between ocular chloramphenicol and aplastic anaemia – the absolute risk is very low. *Br J Clin Pharmacol*. 1998; **46**: 181–4.

Sheikh A, Hurwitz B. Topical antibiotics for acute bacterial conjunctivitis: Cochrane systematic review and meta-analysis update. *Br J Gen Pract*. 2005; **55**: 962–4.

[11.3.1] Fusidic acid (OTC from optometrist)

Class:	anti-staphylococcal topical antibiotic
Eye drops:	1% in a gel
Dose:	adults and children: apply twice a day
Pack:	5 g
Side-effects:	discomfort on administration; rarely local hypersensitivity reactions
Interactions:	none
Cautions:	avoid wearing contact lenses as they can be discoloured or scratched by crystals in the gel
Selection:	this alternative to chloramphenicol is preferred for people who:

- are pregnant
- have a personal or family history of blood dyscrasias, such as aplastic anaemia
- are intolerant of chloramphenicol
- prefer a twice-a-day treatment for infective conjunctivitis

The disadvantage is that the spectrum of bacteria covered by this antibiotic is narrow compared with chloramphenicol

References

Doughty MJ, Dutton GN. Fusidic acid viscous eyedrops: an evaluation of pharmacodynamics, pharmacokinetics and clinical use for UK optometrists. *Ophthalmic Physiol Opt*. 2006; **26**: 343–61.

Rietveld RP, Ter Riet G, Bindels PJ, *et al*. The treatment of acute infectious conjunctivitis with fusidic acid: a randomised controlled trial. *Br J Gen Pract*. 2005; **55**: 924–30.

[11.4.2] Azelastine eye drops (OTC adults and children 12 years and over)

Class:	topical antihistamine
Eye drops:	0.05%
Dose:	adults and children over 4 years: 1 drop to each eye twice a day, increasing to 4 times if necessary
Pack:	8 mL
$t_{1/2}$:	plasma elimination 20 h, of the active metabolite 45 h, but the clinical effect is local
Side-effects:	transient stinging, occasionally bitter taste in mouth
Interactions:	none
Cautions:	discard 1 month after opening, avoid using in pregnancy and breastfeeding
Selection:	antihistamine eye drops can provide relief of symptoms considerably faster than a mast cell stabiliser, such as sodium cromoglicate. Azelastine has a low risk of side-effects and is licensed for both seasonal and perennial conjunctivitis. There is no evidence of safety in pregnancy or breastfeeding – if treatment is essential, an oral antihistamine such as promethazine (in pregnancy) or cetirizine (in lactation) would be preferable

References

Bielory L, Lien KW, Bigelsen S. Efficacy and tolerability of newer antihistamines in the treatment of allergic conjunctivitis. *Drugs*. 2005; **65**: 215–28.

Owen CG, Shah A, Henshaw K, *et al*. Topical treatments for seasonal allergic conjunctivitis: systematic review and meta-analysis of efficacy and effectiveness. *Br J Gen Pract*. 2004; **54**: 451–6.

UKMi Central. *Drugs in Lactation*. 2011. Available at: www.ukmicentral.nhs.uk/drugpreg/antihistamines.asp (accessed 26 August 2011).

[11.4.2] Sodium cromoglicate eye drops (OTC)

Class:	preventative anti-inflammatory – mast cell stabiliser
Eye drops:	2%
Dose:	adults and children: 1 drop four times a day
Pack:	13.5 mL
Side-effects:	transient stinging, avoid wearing soft contact lenses during treatment
Interactions:	none
Caution:	discard 1 month after opening
Selection:	sodium cromoglicate inhibits the release of histamine from mast cells responding to an allergen, so its role is in preventing symptoms rather than controlling them once they have started. It may take several weeks or even months to achieve maximal effect. It is considered safe in pregnancy and breastfeeding

Reference

Prodigy. *Clinical topic: seasonal or perennial allergic conjunctivitis.* 2011. Available at: http://prodigy.clarity.co.uk/conjunctivitis_allergic/management/scenario_seasonal_or_perennial_allergic_conjunctivitis (accessed 28 November 2011).

[11.8.1] Viscotears® (OTC)

Class:	tear replacement
Liquid gel:	polyacrylic acid carbomer 980, 0.2%
Dose:	use as needed, usually 1 drop 4 times a day
Pack:	10 g
Side-effects:	rarely, mild, transient eye irritation, eyelid swelling
Interactions:	none
Cautions:	discard 1 month after opening; unsuitable for use with contact lenses
Selection:	hypromellose is the most commonly used product, but requires frequent administration. Products containing carbomers are longer-acting. As Viscotears does not contain benzalkonium chloride, it has a low risk of causing hypersensitivity reactions, and if it does, there is a preservative-free version available. If the patient does not obtain adequate relief with this preparation, it is worth trying an alternative listed in the *BNF*

References

Doughty MJ, Glavin S. Efficacy of different dry eye treatments with artificial tears or ocular lubricants: a systematic review. *Ophthalmic Physiol Opt.* 2009; **29**: 573–83.

Prodigy. *Clinical topic: Dry eye syndrome.* 2011. Available at: http://prodigy.clarity.co.uk/dry_eye_syndrome (accessed 11 August 2011).

Versura P, Maltarello MC, Stecher F, *et al.* Dry eye before and after therapy with hydroxypropyl methylcellulose. Ultrastructural and cytochemical study in 20 patients. *Ophthalmologica.* 1989; **198**: 152–62.

Ear, nose and oropharynx

[12.1.1] EarCalm® (OTC)

Class:	antibacterial and antifungal topical solution
Spray:	acetic acid 2%
Dose:	adults and children over 12 years: 1 spray into affected ear(s) at least 3 times a day, up to a maximum of 1 spray every 2–3 h, until 2 days after symptoms have resolved but no longer than 1 week
Pack:	5 mL
Side-effects:	transient stinging
Interactions:	none
Cautions:	manufacturer advises treatment for children under 12 years only on medical advice
Selection:	as this preparation is available OTC, many people successfully treat themselves for this condition on the advice of their pharmacist, without any need for swabs to be taken. The advantage of simple acetic acid is that it is an antiseptic with a wide range of mild activity against both bacteria and fungi, but without the risk of either sensitisation to an antibiotic, or fungal superinfection caused by topical steroids. The disadvantage of this preparation is that it is not as effective as a corticosteroid plus either acetic acid or antibacterial. There is no steroid/acetic acid preparation marketed in the UK without an antibiotic, so that option is currently unavailable. For more inflamed cases of otitis externa, a topical steroid/antibacterial combination and/or oral antibiotic is recommended

References

Rowlands S, Devalia H, Smith C, *et al*. Otitis externa in UK general practice: a survey using the UK General Practice Research Database. *Br J Gen Pract*. 2001; **51**: 533–8.

Van Balen FA, Smit WM, Zuithoff NP, *et al*. Clinical efficacy of three common treatments in acute otitis externa in primary care: randomised controlled trial. *BMJ*. 2003; **327**: 1201–5.

[12.1.1] Otosporin®

Class:	bactericidal antibiotics and corticosteroid topical solution
Ear drops:	hydrocortisone 1%, neomycin 3400 units/mL, polymyxin B 10 000 units/mL
Dose:	3 drops into the ear 3 times a day
Pack:	5, 10 mL
Side-effects:	occasional sensitivity reactions, with an increased risk in patients with chronic otitis externa or venous disease such as varicose eczema or ulceration. The drops may sting on application
Interactions:	none
Cautions:	if the tympanic membrane is perforated, consult doctor (who may consider an alternative topical antibiotic such as ofloxacin). Avoid prolonged use: usually 1 week is sufficient. If the condition fails to respond or gets worse, take a swab to identify infections not affected by the antibiotics in Otosporin, such as fungal, but also stop the Otosporin in case the patient has developed a sensitivity to it. Advise the patient not to wash the ear canal using soap or shampoo, as this could inactivate the antibiotics as well as exacerbating the underlying eczema
Selection:	the two antibiotics in this preparation are active against a wide range of bacteria, including *Pseudomonas*. Swabs from infected cases of otitis externa in primary care frequently grow this organism. The fact that patients present more often in the summer months with *Pseudomonas* infection after swimming in pools suggests that this microorganism is more than a bystander. Advise the patient not to try to clean the ear canals after recovery, as the wax has antibacterial properties that can help defend against recurrence

References

Hajjartabar M. Poor-quality water in swimming pools associated with a substantial risk of otitis externa due to *Pseudomonas aeruginosa*. *Water Sci Technol*. 2004; **50**: 63–7.

Lum CL, Jeyanthi S, Prepageran N, *et al*. Antibacterial and antifungal properties of human cerumen. *J Laryngol Otol*. 2009; **123**: 375–8.

[12.1.1] Locorten-Vioform®

Class:	antibacterial, antifungal and corticosteroid topical solution
Ear drops:	flumetasone pivalate 0.02%, clioquinol 1%
Dose:	adults and children over 2 years: 2–3 drops into the ear twice daily for 7–10 days
Pack:	7.5 mL
Side-effects:	stains skin, hair and materials such as pillowcases and clothing brown. Occasionally local irritation or rash. Rarely hypersensitivity reactions may occur. Treatment should be discontinued if patients experience severe irritation or sensitisation
Cautions:	avoid if the patient is allergic to iodine. If the tympanic membrane is perforated, consult doctor (who may consider an alternative topical antibiotic such as ofloxacin)
Selection:	the advantage of this preparation is that it targets both fungal and bacterial infections and avoids the use of neomycin, which is ototoxic in the presence of perforation and the most common reason for a patient developing sensitivity to antibiotic ear drops. It requires only 2 doses per day. The disadvantages of Locorten-Vioform are that it is ineffective against *Pseudomonas* and patients may find the potential to stain hair and materials unacceptable

References

Agius AM, Reid AP, Hamilton C. Patient compliance with short-term topical aural antibiotic therapy. *Clin Otolaryngol Allied Sci*. 1994; **19**(2): 138–41.

Sander R. Otitis externa: a practical guide to treatment and prevention. *Am Fam Physician*. 2001; **63**(5): 927–36.

[12.1.1] Otomize®

Class:	mixed antibacterials and corticosteroid topical solution
Spray:	dexamethasone 0.1%, neomycin 3250 units/mL, glacial acetic acid 2%
Dose:	1 metered spray into the ear 3 times a day
Pack:	5 mL
Side-effects:	occasional sensitivity reactions, with an increased risk in patients with chronic otitis externa or eczema
Interactions:	none
Cautions:	if previous perforation, consult doctor (who may consider an alternative topical antibiotic such as ofloxacin). Avoid prolonged use: usually 1 week is sufficient. If the condition fails to respond or gets worse, take a swab to identify infections not affected by the antibacterials in Otomize, such as fungi, but also stop the Otomize in case the patient has developed sensitivity to it. Advise the patient not to wash the ear canal using soap or shampoo, as this could inactivate the antibacterials as well as exacerbating the underlying eczema
Selection:	the spray delivery of Otomize provides a more accurate dose than self-administered drops, may be more effective and is often preferred by patients. The options of different topical treatments for otitis externa can be summarised as follows:

- EarCalm: low risk of complications but less effective, available OTC
- Otosporin: first-line after swimming, hot tubs, or with vivid green exudate from the ear
- Locorten-Vioform: broad activity including antifungal, staining may be unacceptable
- Otomize: more effective than EarCalm, acceptable, but no anti-pseudomonal as in Otosporin

References

Connolly AA, Picozzi GL, Browning GG. Randomized trial of neomycin/dexamethasone spray vs drop preparation for the treatment of active chronic mucosal otitis media. *Clin Otolaryngol.* 1997; **22**: 529–31.

Johnston MN, Flook EP, Mehta D, *et al.* Prospective randomised single-blind controlled trial of glacial acetic acid versus glacial acetic acid, neomycin sulphate and dexamethasone spray in otitis externa and infected mastoid cavities. *Clin Otolaryngol.* 2006; **31**: 504–7.

Lancaster J, Mathews J, Williams RS, *et al.* Comparison of compliance between topical aural medications. *Clin Otolaryngol.* 2003; **28**: 331–4.

[12.2.1] Azelastine nasal spray (OTC adults and children 5 years and over)

Class:	topical antihistamine
Nasal spray:	140 µg per dose
Dose:	adults and children over 5 years: 1 spray into each nostril twice a day
Pack:	22 mL
$t_{1/2}$:	plasma elimination 20 h, of the active metabolite 45 h, but the clinical effect is local
Side-effects:	transient stinging, occasionally bitter taste in mouth
Interactions:	none
Cautions:	avoid using in pregnancy and breastfeeding
Selection:	for intermittent symptoms of rhinitis, an intranasal antihistamine provides treatment as required. If symptoms are persistent, a corticosteroid spray used regularly during the allergic period is more suitable. Azelastine offers better control of rhinitis that an oral antihistamine, but people who also have allergic conjunctivitis might prefer an oral antihistamine to treat both conditions. There is no evidence of safety of azelastine in pregnancy or breastfeeding – if treatment is essential an oral antihistamine such as pro-methazine (in pregnancy) or cetirizine (in lactation) would be preferable

References

Prodigy. *Clinical topic: Allergic rhinitis*. 2011. Available at: http://prodigy.clarity.co.uk/allergic_rhinitis (accessed 11 August 2011).

Scadding GK, Durham SR, Mirakianz R, *et al*. BSACI guidelines for the management of allergic and non-allergic rhinitis. *Clin Exp Allergy*. 2008; **38**: 19–42.

UKMi Central. *Drugs in Lactation*. 2011. Available at: www.ukmicentral.nhs.uk/drugpreg/antihistamines.asp (accessed 26 August 2011).

[12.2.1] Rhinocort Aqua® (OTC)

Class:	corticosteroid
Nasal spray:	budesonide 64 µg per spray
Dose:	adults and children over 12 years: initially 2 sprays to each nostril every morning; when symptoms are controlled, reduce to 1 spray
Pack:	120-spray unit
$t_{1/2}$:	plasma elimination 3 h, but the clinical effect is local
Side-effects:	dry nose or throat, epistaxis, altered smell or taste; rarely ulceration of the nasal septum, bronchospasm, headache, raised intraocular pressure or glaucoma, growth retardation in children, allergic reactions
Interactions:	none
Cautions:	untreated nasal infection, recent nasal surgery, pulmonary tuberculosis, duration of treatment normally limited to 3 months, avoid in pregnancy and breastfeeding
Selection:	with no evidence to suggest superiority of any particular topical steroid for hay fever, the selection is made on the basis of convenience to the patient, with once-daily dosing and low cost. There will be some benefit on the first day of use, but this increases over the next few days, so ideally patients should start treatment 1 week before their hay fever season starts. Reducing the allergic response in the nose may also reduce inflammation elsewhere in the respiratory tract, which is particularly helpful in asthma. About a third of the nasal dose is absorbed, but the dose of corticosteroid is so low that systemic side-effects are extremely rare

References

Kim KT, Rabinovitch N, Uryniak T, *et al*. Effect of budesonide aqueous nasal spray on hypothalamic-pituitary-adrenal axis function in children with allergic rhinitis. *Ann Allergy Asthma Immunol*. 2004; **93**: 61–7.

Scichilone N, Arrigo R, Paterno A, *et al*. The effect of intranasal corticosteroids on asthma control and quality of life in allergic rhinitis with mild asthma. *J Asthma*. 2011; **48**: 41–7.

Stanaland BE. Once-daily budesonide aqueous nasal spray for allergic rhinitis: a review. *Clin Ther*. 2004; **26**: 473–92.

[12.2.2] Sodium chloride: Stérimar® (OTC)

Class:	topical nasal decongestant
Spray:	purified sea water, hypertonic, isotonic
Dose:	adults and children over 3 years: 2–6 sprays of hypertonic into each nostril per day
	children 3 months–3 years: 2–6 sprays of isotonic into each nostril per day
Pack:	50 mL
Side-effects:	none
Interactions:	none
Cautions:	none
Selection:	helps to liquefy nasal mucous secretions

References

Papsin B, McTavish A. Saline nasal irrigation: its role as an adjunct treatment. *Can Fam Physician*. 2003; **49**: 168–73.

Patient UK. *Blocked Nose in Babies (Snuffles)*. 2011. Available at: www.patient.co.uk/showdoc/23069191/ (accessed 14 August 2011).

www.sterimar.com/en

[12.2.2] Warm moist air inhalation

Class: topical nasal decongestant

Liquid: very hot water

Dose: inhale 3 or 4 times a day with a towel over the head

Pack: not applicable

Side-effects: only the risk of scalds from the hot water

Interactions: none

Cautions: a hot shower would be safer, but if using a bowl then place it in a basin so that it cannot be tipped over

Selection: helps to liquefy nasal mucous secretions. Adding aromatic oils may make the experience more soothing

References

Akhavani MA, Baker RH. Steam inhalation treatment for children. *Br J Gen Pract*. 2005; 55(516): 557.

Singh M, Singh M. Heated, humidified air for the common cold. *Cochrane Database Syst Rev*. 2011; 5: CD001728.

[12.2.2] Ephedrine nasal drops (OTC)

Class:	topical nasal decongestant
Drops:	0.5%
Dose:	adults and children over 12 years: 1–2 drops into each nostril 3–4 times daily when required for up to 1 week
Pack:	10 mL
$t_{1/2}$:	3–6 h
Side-effects:	the main risk is from use over 1 week, when the medication becomes less effective (tolerance) and causes rebound congestion on stopping. Local irritation, nausea, headache, possible cardiovascular effects such as palpitations and tachycardia
Interactions:	theophylline, monoamine oxidase inhibitor antidepressants. There are other theoretical interactions with a wide range of medications listed in Appendix 1 of the *BNF* under Sympathomimetics, but the amount of ephedrine absorbed from the nose is too low to make such interactions likely
Cautions:	avoid in unstable cardiovascular disease including uncontrolled hypertension; limit use to 1 week. Be careful to prescribe the correct strength, as other preparations may be 'specials' which are extremely expensive
Selection:	less likely to cause rebound congestion than alternative adrenaline-like nasal decongestants. The amount of drug absorbed and risk of generalised adrenaline-like effects is low, but not without some risk, so only prescribe if the benefit is thought to outweigh the slight risk. Many patients find nasal drops difficult to use correctly, so a decongestant spray may be preferable, and there are many varieties available OTC

References

Caravati EM. Reconsidering the safety of over-the-counter decongestants. *Ann Emerg Med*. 2005; **45**: 217–18.

Joint Formulary Committee. *Topical Nasal Decongestants: British National Formulary*. (Notes to section 12.2.2.) Available at: http://bnf.org/bnf/bnf/current/5656.htm (accessed 14 August 2011).

Zhang L, Han D, Song X, *et al*. Effects of ephedrine on human nasal ciliary beat frequency. *J Otorhinolaryngol Relat Spec*. 2008; **70**: 91–6.

[12.3.1] Benzydamine (OTC)

Class:	anti-inflammatory analgesic
Oral rinse/ spray:	benzydamine hydrochloride 0.15%
Dose:	use every 1.5–3 h for up to 1 week

oral rinse:
adults and children over 12 years: rinse or gargle using 15 mL

spray:
adults and children over 12 years: 4–8 sprays onto affected area
children 6–12 years: 4 sprays onto affected area
under 6 years: 1 spray per 4 kg body weight (maximum 4)

Pack:	300 mL oral rinse, 30 mL spray
Side-effects:	occasional oral numbness or stinging sensations (dilute the rinse with an equal volume of water if stinging occurs); very rarely hypersensitivity reactions
Interactions:	none
Cautions:	none
Selection:	benzydamine is an anti-inflammatory analgesic that inhibits prostaglandin synthesis, similar to the action of NSAIDs, effective locally but without significant systemic effects

References

Cingi C, Songu M, Ural A, *et al.* Effect of chlorhexidine gluconate and benzydamine hydrochloride mouth spray on clinical signs and quality of life of patients with streptococcal tonsillopharyngitis: multicentre, prospective, randomised, double-blinded, placebo-controlled study. *J Laryngol Otol.* 2011; **11**: 1–6.

Cingi C, Songu M, Ural A, *et al.* Effects of chlorhexidine/benzydamine mouth spray on pain and quality of life in acute viral pharyngitis: a prospective, randomized, double-blind, placebo-controlled, multicenter study. *Ear Nose Throat J.* 2010; **89**: 546–9.

Matthews RW, Scully CM, Levers BG, *et al.* Clinical evaluation of benzydamine, chlorhexidine, and placebo mouthwashes in the management of recurrent aphthous stomatitis. *Oral Surg Oral Med Oral Pathol.* 1987; **63**: 189–91.

Wethington JF. Double-blind study of benzydamine hydrochloride, a new treatment for sore throat. *Clin Ther.* 1985; **7**: 641–6.

[12.3.1] Hydrocortisone mucoadhesive buccal tablets (OTC)

Class:	corticosteroid for oral ulceration
Mucoadhesive buccal tablets:	2.5 mg
Dose:	adults and children over 12 years: 1 tablet dissolved over the ulcer 4 times a day
Pack:	20
Side-effects:	local discomfort, exacerbation of local infection, oral thrush
Interactions:	none
Cautions:	consider the differential diagnosis carefully. Ask about other symptoms and whether there are cutaneous lesions elsewhere. Important causes include oral herpes, cancer, inflammatory bowel disease (e.g. Crohn's disease), autoimmune disease (e.g. Behçet's disease), food allergy and vitamin deficiencies. Be suspicious of an underlying cause of any ulcer present for over 3 weeks
Selection:	hydrocortisone is the corticosteroid available in a suitable formulation for relieving symptoms of aphthous ulcers. It does not reduce the likelihood of recurrence or address any underlying cause

References

Scully C, Porter S. Oral mucosal disease: recurrent aphthous stomatitis. *Br J Oral Maxillofac Surg.* 2008; **46**: 198–206.

Tilliss TSI, McDowell JD. Differential diagnosis: is it herpes or aphthous? *J Contemp Dent Pract.* 2002; **3**: 1–15.

Wardhana, Datau EA. Recurrent aphthous stomatitis caused by food allergy. *Acta Med Indones.* 2010; **42**: 236–40.

Wray D, Ferguson MM, Hutcheon AW, *et al*. Nutritional deficiencies in recurrent aphthae. *J Oral Pathol Med.* 1978; **7**: 418–23.

[12.3.2] Miconazole oral gel (OTC 15 g for age over 4 months)

Class:	imidazole antifungal
Oral gel:	24 mg/mL
Dose:	(all after food and, whenever practical, retained near the lesions before swallowing)
	adults and children over 12 years: 5–10 mL in the mouth, 4 times a day
	children 6–12 years: 5 mL in the mouth, 4 times a day
	2–6 years: 5 mL in the mouth, twice a day
	1 month–2 years (unlicensed use under 4 months): 2.5 mL smeared around the mouth, twice a day
	under 1 month (unlicensed use): 1 mL 2–4 times daily smeared around the mouth after feeds
Pack:	15, 80 g
Side-effects:	nausea and vomiting, diarrhoea (with long-term treatment); rarely allergic reactions; isolated reports of hepatitis
Interactions:	sufficient absorption of miconazole oral gel occurs to interact with other medication including **warfarin**, and because it inhibits the action of liver enzymes that eliminate many drugs, there are many potential interactions. For a list, see Appendix 1 in the *BNF* under 'Antifungals, Imidazole'
Cautions:	avoid in liver disease
Selection:	miconazole oral gel is recommended for treating oral fungal infections in children under 2 years of age. Trial evidence indicates that it is safe and more effective than nystatin. Children of this age are unlikely to be taking other medication, so this avoids the problem of drug interactions. Older children who are otherwise healthy rarely get oral candidal infection. Treatment should continue until 48 h after lesions have resolved. Reports of babies briefly choking on the gel resulted in the change of license to over 4 months of age. The risk is very low, but if prescribing for this age group advise the parent to apply the gel directly to the inner surfaces of the baby's mouth where they can see or feel where it is going, and not to try to treat the baby by applying the gel to mother's nipples before a feed

References

De Vries TW, Wewerinke ME, De Langen JJ. Near asphyxiation of a neonate due to miconazole oral gel. *Ned Tijdschr Geneeskd.* 2004; **148**: 1598–600.

Hoppe JE. Treatment of oropharyngeal candidiasis in immunocompetent infants: a randomized multicenter study of miconazole gel vs. nystatin suspension. The Antifungals Study Group. *Paediatr Infect Dis J.* 1997; **16**: 288–93.

Hoppe JE, Hahn H. Randomized comparison of two nystatin oral gels with miconazole oral gel for the treatment of oral thrush in infants. Antimycotics Study Group. *Infection.* 1996; **24**: 136–9.

[12.3.4] Chlorhexidine (OTC)

Class:	antiseptic
Oral rinse/ spray:	chlorhexidine gluconate 0.2%
Dose:	oral rinse:
	adults and children over 12 years: rinse mouth with 10 mL for about 1 minute twice a day, then spit out (not intended to be swallowed)
	oral spray:
	adults and children (age range not specified – on medical advice under 12 years): up to 12 actuations of the spray to ulcer(s) twice daily
Pack:	300 mL oral rinse, 60 mL spray
Side-effects:	chlorhexidine has been associated with bitter taste, brown staining of teeth and tongue, and nausea, but these effects are less likely with the limited amount required to cover an oral ulcer with the spray compared with a mouthwash. Oral irritation (dilute the rinse with an equal volume of water if this occurs), taste disturbance; rarely parotid swelling
Interactions:	leave at least 30 minutes between using toothpaste and chlorhexidine as the ingredients may be incompatible
Cautions:	none
Selection:	superficial infection may play a part in the symptoms caused by aphthous ulcers. Chlorhexidine is a general antiseptic with limited evidence of effectiveness in reducing the severity, duration and incidence of oral ulceration

References

Addy M, Carpenter R, Roberts WR. Management of recurrent aphthous ulceration. A trial of chlorhexidine gluconate gel. *Br Dent J*. 1976; **141**: 118–20.

Clinical Evidence. *Aphthous Ulcers: chlorhexidine and similar agents*. 2004. Available at: http://clinicalevidence.bmj.com

Miles DA, Bricker SL, Razmus TF, *et al*. Triamcinolone acetonide versus chlorhexidine for treatment of recurrent stomatitis. *Oral Surg Oral Med Oral Pathol*. 1993; **75**: 397–402.

Prodigy. *Aphthous ulcers*. 2011. Available at: http://prodigy.clarity.co.uk/aphthous_ulcer (accessed 11 August 2011).

Skin

[13.2.1] Aqueous cream; emulsifying ointment; hydrous ointment; paraffin, yellow soft BP; Cetraben®; E45® lotion (OTC)

Class:	emollients
Dose:	apply in the direction of hair growth as frequently as necessary, or add 1–3 capfuls to bath
Pack:	500 g cream/ointment; 100 g paraffin; 50, 150, 500 g pump dispenser of Cetraben; 500 mL pump dispenser of E45 lotion
Side-effects:	rarely sensitisation to an excipient in an emollient (consult the listed excipients in the table in *MIMS* to help in choosing an alternative)
Interactions:	none
Cautions:	fire hazard, can make the surface of a bath slippery
Selection:	emollients hydrate the skin and are useful in all dry or scaling disorders. Light creams are only useful as a soap substitute, where thicker ointments can be applied directly to rehydrate and soothe the skin. The choice is mainly a matter of patient preference. Initially prescribe small amounts and if necessary try a variety of products until the patient's preference is established, and then prescribe enough by consulting the guide at the start of section 13.1.2 in the *BNF*. A pump dispenser reduces the chance of infection in the unused product, and can be helpful to a parent who needs to hold a small child with one hand, or a patient who would have difficulty with a normal tube or tub

Reference

Berth-Jones J, Graham-Brown RAC. How useful are soap substitutes? *J Dermatol Treat.* 1992; 3: 9–11.

[13.2.1.1] QV® bath oil; Hydromol® bath and shower emollient (OTC)

Class: emollient bath additives

Dose: add to bath

QV
adults: 10 mL
child: 7 mL
infant: 4 mL

Hydromol
adults: 1–3 capfuls
infant: 0.5–2 capfuls

Pack: QV bath oil 200, 500 mL; Hydromol 350, 500, 1000 mL

Side-effects: can make the surface of a bath slippery; rarely sensitisation

Interactions: none

Cautions: none

Selection: addition of emollients to the bath may be a practical way to hydrate extensive area of dry skin, but there are no published randomised controlled trials on their use in atopic eczema, so they should not replace directly applied emollients. Use in the shower is likely to be less effective, because of the shorter duration of contact. The choice is largely based on patients' preference and cost. The cost varies between brands, with these two being inexpensive at about 8p per bath or shower. Oils can make the bath slippery, difficult to clean and leave a slightly sticky residue on facecloths. In contrast, emulsions mix with the bath water. Hydromol bath and shower emollient is a water-dispersible bath additive resulting in an emulsion of dispersed oils together with a homogenised film on the surface

References

[No authors listed]. Bath emollients for atopic eczema: why use them? *Drug Ther Bull*. 2007; **45**: 73–5.

Tarr A, Iheanacho I. Should we use bath emollients for atopic eczema? *BMJ*. 2009; **339**: b4273.

[13.2.2] Metanium® (OTC)

Class:	barrier
Ointment:	titanium dioxide 20%, titanium peroxide 5%, titanium salicylate 3%
Dose:	apply with each nappy change
Pack:	30 g
Side-effects:	none
Interactions:	none
Cautions:	none
Selection:	an effective barrier that does not contain excipients likely to cause any skin sensitisation

References

Ereaux LP. Clinical observations on the use of titanium salts in the treatment of dermatitis. *Can Med Assoc J.* 1955; 73: 47.

Prodigy. *Nappy Rash.* 2011. Available at: http://prodigy.clarity.co.uk/nappy_rash/management/scenario_management/treatment - -380192 (accessed 15 August 2011).

[13.3] Crotamiton (OTC)

Class:	antipruritic
Cream or lotion:	10%
Dose:	adults and children over 3 years: apply 2–3 times daily
	children under 3 years: apply once daily
Pack:	cream 30, 100 g; lotion 100 mL
Side-effects:	skin irritation, contact dermatitis
Interactions:	none
Cautions:	avoid in acute exudative dermatoses or application to damaged skin; manufacturer advises avoid in pregnancy; do not apply near nipples if breastfeeding
Selection:	there are no published comparative trials on the effectiveness of topical antipruritics, but despite this, crotamiton has a long history of use and is often recommended

References

Hara H, Masuda T, Yokoyama A, *et al*. Allergic contact dermatitis due to crotamiton. *Contact Dermatitis*. 2003; **49**: 219.

Johnston G, Sladden M. Scabies: diagnosis and treatment. *BMJ*. 2005; **331**: 619–22.

[13.4] Topical corticosteroids: hydrocortisone 1% (OTC with restrictions) – *mild*; Eumovate®, Betnovate RD® – *moderate*; Betnovate® – *potent*

Class:	topical corticosteroids
Cream or ointment:	various concentrations
Dose:	apply once daily (occasionally twice daily may be required)
Pack:	hydrocortisone 15, 30, 50 g; Eumovate and Betnovate 30, 100 g; Betnovate RD 100 g
Side-effects:	worsening of infection including acne, thinning and potential permanent disfiguring marks of skin with potency greater than hydrocortisone, increased hair growth, perioral dermatitis (papular rash around the mouth in young women), depigmentation; potent preparations used on large areas may be absorbed into the body and cause similar side-effects to oral steroids; rarely sensitisation to an excipient (consult the listed excipients in the table in *MIMS* to help in choosing an alternative)
Interactions:	none
Cautions:	skin infection including acne, do not use moderate or potent corticosteroids on the face, children are more susceptible to side-effects, psoriasis (may rebound or relapse on stopping)
Selection:	topical corticosteroids are helpful in treating dry skin conditions. The general rule is to use none if an emollient will suffice, otherwise to use the mildest effective potency. Some of the therapeutic effect of these preparations is due to the emollient vehicle rather than just the steroid component. Sensitisation to one of the excipients can occur and lead to diagnostic confusion when a dermatitis persists or worsens despite treatment. The risk of skin atrophy when using topical steroids increases with potency, and to a lesser extent the concentration of the steroid. The following mnemonic may help:

Hydrocortisone – Harmless
Eumovate – Easy-going
Betnovate – Beware of skin atrophy
Dermovate – Dangerous

References

[No authors listed]. Topical steroids for atopic dermatitis in primary care. *Drug Ther Bull*. 2003; **41**: 5–8.

Charman CR, Morris AD, Williams HC. Topical corticosteroid phobia in patients with atopic eczema. *Br J Dermatol*. 2000; **142**: 931–6.

National Prescribing Centre. Using topical corticosteroids in general practice. *MeReC Bull*. 1999; **10**: 21–4.

Parneix-Spake A, Goustas P, Green R. Eumovate (clobetasone butyrate) 0.05% cream with its moisturizing emollient base has better healing properties than hydrocortisone 1% cream: a study in nickel-induced contact dermatitis. *J Dermatol Treat*. 2001; **12**: 191–7.

[13.4] Canesten HC® (OTC)

Class:	topical antifungal and corticosteroid
Cream:	clotrimazole 1% and hydrocortisone 1% ointment
Dose:	adults and children: apply twice daily
Pack:	30 g
Side-effects:	*see* hydrocortisone
Interactions:	none
Cautions:	*see* hydrocortisone
Selection:	for simple fungal skin infections, use plain clotrimazole topically (*see* section 13.10.2). If pruritus is troublesome, or the fungal infection is in an eczematous area, the combination of an antifungal agent with a corticosteroid can be helpful. Both clotrimazole and miconazole are the same type of imidazole antifungal agents, so if a fungal infection does not respond to one it will not respond to the other. Terbinafine cream is then a suitable alternative

Reference

Crawford F, Hollis S. Topical treatments for fungal infections of the skin and nails of the foot. *Cochrane Database Syst Rev.* 2007; **3**: CD001434.

[13.6.1] Benzoyl peroxide (OTC)

Class:	topical preparation for acne – sebostatic. Keratolytic, antibacterial activity against *Propionibacterium acnes*
Gel:	2.5%, 5%, 10%
Cream:	4%, 5%
Dose:	adults and children over 12 years: apply thinly 1–2 times daily after washing with soap and water. Continue for at least 6 weeks. Start with the 2.5% gel and only increase the strength if necessary, as there is evidence that this concentration is as effective as higher ones
Pack:	gel 40, 60 g, cream 40 g
Side-effects:	local skin reaction (a mild redness of the skin is to be expected following initial application). Bleaching of clothing or hair on contact
Interactions:	none
Cautions:	avoid contact with eyes, mucous membranes or other areas of sensitive skin
Selection:	mild to moderate acne with comedones responds well to benzoyl peroxide, which has antibacterial activity against the microorganism that causes acne vulgaris. It does not cause bacterial resistance during long-term use. It may be used in pregnancy and breastfeeding

References

Goulden V. Guidelines for the management of acne vulgaris in adolescents. *Paediatr Drugs*. 2003; 5: 301–13.

Purdy S, Deberker D. Acne vulgaris. *Clin Evid (Online)*. 2011; pii: 1714 (accessed 15 August 2011).

[13.6.1] Duac® once daily gel

Class:	topical preparation for acne – sebostatic. Keratolytic, antibacterial activity against *Propionibacterium acnes*
Gel:	benzoyl peroxide 5%, clindamycin 1%
Dose:	adults and children over 12 years: apply once daily in the evening after washing with soap and water for up to 12 weeks
Pack:	25, 50 g
Side-effects:	local skin reaction, bleaching of clothing or hair on contact. If diarrhoea occurs, discontinue and check for *Clostridium difficile*. There have been reports concerning topical clindamycin, but the company say 'In a few susceptible individuals there have been isolated reports of pseudomembraneous colitis or diarrhoea due to other topical treatments containing clindamycin. This is unlikely to occur with Duac Once Daily Gel, as plasma levels have been determined and the percutaneous absorption of clindamycin is clinically negligible'. Worsening of acne has been reported
Interactions:	manufacturer advised against use in combination with topical retinoids (adapalene, isotretinoin, tretinoin) but there are published trials of such a combination
Cautions:	avoid contact with eyes, mucous membranes or other areas of sensitive skin, avoid in pregnancy; caution with history of atopy, ulcerative or antibiotic-associated colitis
Selection:	as the benzoyl peroxide component can prevent the development of resistance, it is useful in combination with antibacterials

References

[No authors listed]. What role for topical antibacterials in acne? *Drug Ther Bull*. 2010; **48**: 141–4.

Ingram JR, Grindlay DJ, Williams HC. Management of acne vulgaris: an evidence-based update. *Clin Exp Dermatol*. 2010; **35**: 351–4.

[13.6.1] Azelaic acid

Class:	topical preparation for acne – sebostatic. Keratolytic, antibacterial activity against *Propionibacterium acnes*
Gel:	15%
Cream:	20%
Dose:	adults and children over 12 years: lightly massage into the skin twice daily after washing with soap and water (if sensitive skin, once daily for the first week)
Pack:	30 g (enough to treat the entire facial skin for 1 month)
Side-effects:	local skin reaction, occasionally skin discolouration, very rarely photosensitisation
Interactions:	none
Cautions:	discontinue and consider an alternative treatment if no improvement occurs after 1 month. Avoid contact with eyes, mucous membranes or other areas of sensitive skin
Selection:	azelaic acid is an alternative to benzoyl peroxide that is rated as 'well tolerated' or 'very well tolerated' by 96% of patients. It is almost as effective. Several months' treatment may be required, but the manufacturer of the cream advises no longer than one year

References

Gollnick HP, Graupe K, Zaumseil RP. Azelaic acid 15% gel in the treatment of acne vulgaris. Combined results of two double-blind clinical comparative studies. *J Dtsch Dermatol Ges.* 2004; **2**: 841–7.

Thiboutot D. Versatility of azelaic acid 15% gel in treatment of inflammatory acne vulgaris. *J Drugs Dermatol.* 2008; **7**: 13–16.

[13.6.1] Zineryt®

Class:	topical antibacterial with zinc as an aid to skin healing
Solution:	erythromycin 40 mg, zinc acetate 12 mg/mL
Dose:	adults and children: apply twice daily
Pack:	30, 90 mL
Side-effects:	rare local skin reactions
Interactions:	none
Cautions:	avoid if the patient is allergic to the ingredients
Selection:	this preparation has a broad spectrum of use in adults and children, pregnancy and breastfeeding. Side-effects are rare, making it a good choice for people with sensitive skin. The addition of zinc is to aid skin healing. The disadvantage of using a topical antibacterial is the possibility of inducing resistance

References

Habbema L, Koopmans B, Menke HE, *et al.* A 4% erythromycin and zinc combination (Zineryt) versus 2% erythromycin (Eryderm) in acne vulgaris: a randomized, double-blind comparative study. *Br J Dermatol.* 1989; **121**: 497–502.

Langner A, Sheehan-Dare R, Layton A. A randomized, single-blind comparison of topical clindamycin + benzoyl peroxide (Duac) and erythromycin + zinc acetate (Zineryt) in the treatment of mild to moderate facial acne vulgaris. *J Eur Acad Dermatol Venereol.* 2007; **21**: 311–19.

[13.6.1] Tretinoin

Class:	topical retinoid
Gel:	0.01%, 0.025%
Dose:	adults: apply thinly 1–2 times daily for at least 6 weeks. Start with lower-strength preparation.
	children: manufacturer advises not for children
Pack:	60 g
Side-effects:	local skin reactions including temporary colour changes (a mild redness of the skin is to be expected following initial application); eye irritation; increased susceptibility to sunburn
Interactions:	other topical treatments may interact
Cautions:	**avoid in pregnancy, rosacea,** perioral dermatitis, or if the patient or family member has had a cutaneous epithelioma (non-melanoma skin cancer, e.g. basal cell or squamous cell carcinoma); do not apply to areas of eczema. Advise the patient not to sunbathe, use sunlamps, waxing, exfoliants or dying cosmetic preparations on the area of application
Selection:	tretinoin is the acid form of vitamin A. It is useful for treating acne with oily skin. Improvement may take 6–8 weeks to develop, after which the frequency of application can be reduced. There is no risk of inducing bacterial resistance as this is not an antibacterial agent. Women of childbearing age should use effective contraception because oral tretinoin is known to be teratogenic. The *BNF* states that oral progestogen-only contraceptives are *not* considered adequately effective in this respect

References

Bozzo P, Chua-Gocheco A, Einarson A. Safety of skin care products during pregnancy. *Can Fam Physician*. 2011; **57**: 665–7.

Thielitz A, Gollnick H. Topical retinoids in acne vulgaris: update on efficacy and safety. *Am J Clin Dermatol*. 2008; **9**: 369–81.

[13.7] Salactol® (OTC)

Class: topical treatment for warts

Paint: salicylic acid 16.7%, lactic acid 16.7%

Dose: adults and children: apply daily

Pack: 10 mL

Side-effects: local irritation, sensitisation

Interactions: none

Cautions: keep away from the eyes and mucous membranes, flammable

Selection: the limited evidence that is available on the topical treatment of warts suggests salicylic acid is the best option

References

Gibbs S, Harvey I. Topical treatments for cutaneous warts. *Cochrane Database Syst Rev*. 2006; **3**: CD001781.

Kwok CS, Holland R, Gibbs S. Efficacy of topical treatments for cutaneous warts: a meta-analysis and pooled analysis of randomized controlled trials. *Br J Dermatol*. 2011; **165**: 233–46.

[13.9] Ketoconazole shampoo (OTC)

Class:	imidazole antifungal
Shampoo:	ketoconazole 2%
Dose:	adults and children: use twice weekly for up to 4 weeks
Pack:	120 mL
Side-effects:	rarely local irritation; rarely oily or dry hair; discolouration of previously dyed or grey hair; alopecia
Interactions:	none
Cautions:	avoid contact with eyes
Selection:	seborrhoeic dermatitis of the scalp ranges from mild (dandruff) to severe (when expert advice from a dermatologist is advisable). Shampoos, readily available OTC, containing antimicrobial agents such as zinc pyrithione (e.g. Head & Shoulders® anti-dandruff shampoo) and selenium disulphide (e.g. Selsun®) may help, but ketoconazole shampoo is more effective at treating severe cases than zinc pyrithione, just as effective as selenium and better tolerated

References

Danby FW, Maddin WS, Margesson LJ, *et al*. A randomized, double-blind, placebo-controlled trial of ketoconazole 2% shampoo versus selenium sulfide 25% shampoo in the treatment of moderate to severe dandruff. *J Am Acad Dermatol*. 1993; **29**: 1008–12.

Piérard-Franchimont C, Goffin V, Decroix J, *et al*. A multicenter randomized trial of ketoconazole 2% and zinc pyrithione 1% shampoos in severe dandruff and seborrheic dermatitis. *Skin Pharmacol Appl Skin Physiol*. 2002; **15**: 434–41.

[13.9] Capasal® (OTC)

Class:	compound scalp treatment
Shampoo:	salicylic acid 0.5%; coconut oil 1.0%; coal tar 1.0%
Dose:	adults and children: use daily if necessary
Pack:	250 mL
Side-effects:	rarely local irritation
Interactions:	none
Cautions:	avoid contact with eyes
Selection:	although traditionally used for cradle cap in children, this shampoo is also useful in dry, scaly scalp conditions such as seborrhoeic eczema, seborrhoeic dermatitis, pityriasis capitis, and psoriasis

Reference

Klaber MR, McKinnon C. Calcipotriol (Dovonex®) scalp solution in the treatment of scalp psoriasis: Comparative efficacy with 1% coal tar/1% coconut oil/0.5% salicylic acid (Capasal®) shampoo, and long-term experience. *J Dermatol Treat.* 2000; **11**: 21–8.

[13.10.1] Sodium fusidate

Class:	anti-staphylococcal topical antibiotic
Ointment:	2%
Dose:	adults and children: apply 3–4 times a day
Pack:	15, 30 g
Side-effects:	rarely local hypersensitivity reactions
Interactions:	none
Cautions:	avoid contact with eyes
Selection:	this narrow-spectrum antibiotic is very effective against staphylococcal infections. The Cochrane Review of treatment for impetigo concluded that this topical agent is better than oral antibiotics for people with limited disease, and possibly even for those with more extensive disease. We know of no comparative study between fusidic acid cream and sodium fusidate ointment, but it seems more appropriate to use the salt than the acid on areas of skin that are likely to be inflamed and sore. The ointment can also be used to treat angular cheilitis (inflammation of the corners of the lips, which become cracked and sore)

Reference

Koning S, Verhagen AP, van Suijlekom-Smit LWA, *et al*. Interventions for impetigo. *Cochrane Database Syst Rev*. 2004; **2**: CD003261.

[13.10.2] Clotrimazole (OTC)

Class:	imidazole antifungal
All formulations:	clotrimazole 1%
Dose:	adults and children: apply 2–3 times daily
Pack:	cream: 20, 50 g
	powder: 30 g
	liquid: 20 mL
	spray: 40 mL
Side-effects:	rarely local irritation
Interactions:	may cause damage to latex contraceptives
Cautions:	none
Selection:	for simple fungal skin infections, use plain clotrimazole topically. If pruritus is troublesome, or the fungal infection is in an eczematous area, the combination of an antifungal agent with a corticosteroid can be helpful (*see* section 13.4). Both clotrimazole and miconazole are the same type of imidazole antifungal agents, so if a fungal infection does not respond to one it will not respond to the other. Terbinafine cream is then a suitable alternative. For seborrhoeic dermatitis of the scalp, use ketoconazole shampoo

Reference

Crawford F, Hollis S. Topical treatments for fungal infections of the skin and nails of the foot. *Cochrane Database Syst Rev.* 2007; **3**: CD001434.

[13.10.2] Terbinafine (OTC)

Class:	allylamine antifungal
Cream:	1%
Dose:	adults (unlicensed for use in children): apply 1–2 times a day, for 1 week for fungal infections of the feet, 2 weeks if elsewhere
Pack:	15, 30 g
Side-effects:	redness, itching or stinging occasionally occur at the site of application; however, treatment rarely has to be discontinued for this reason. This must be distinguished from allergic reactions, which are rare but require discontinuation
Interactions:	none
Cautions:	avoid contact with eyes, avoid in pregnancy and breastfeeding
Selection:	this broad-spectrum antifungal agent is a useful alternative to clotrimazole because cross-resistance is unusual. Terbinafine can be applied less often and for a shorter course. The Cochrane Review concluded: 'The most cost-effective strategy is first to treat with azoles or undecenoic acid and to use allylamines only if that fails'

Reference

Crawford F, Hollis S. Topical treatments for fungal infections of the skin and nails of the foot. *Cochrane Database Syst Rev.* 2007; 3: CD001434.

[13.10.3] Aciclovir (OTC)

Class:	topical antiviral
Cream:	aciclovir 5%
Dose:	for cold sores
	adults and children: apply every 4 h (5 times a day omitting the night-time) for 5 days at the first sign of an attack, continuing for a further 5 days if the lesions have not completely healed
Pack:	2, 10 g
Side-effects:	transient stinging or burning; occasionally erythema or drying of the skin, sensitivity to excipients
Interactions:	none (interactions listed in the *BNF* apply to tablets and infusions, not the cream)
Cautions:	avoid contact with eyes and mucous membranes, limited data in pregnancy and breastfeeding – but not known to be harmful
Selection:	aciclovir interferes with viral DNA synthesis. It is used topically to treat cold sores, but does not eradicate the virus. Standard advice is that the cream needs to be applied as soon as the first symptom appears, and although this gives the best chance of speedy resolution, the cream is still partially effective if it is applied later. Prophylaxis with topical agents is not effective

References

Spruance SL, Kriesel JD. Treatment of herpes simplex labialis. *Herpes*. 2002; **9**: 64–9.

Spruance SL, Nett R, Marbury T, *et al*. Acyclovir cream for treatment of herpes simplex labialis: results of two randomized, double-blind, vehicle-controlled, multicenter clinical trials. *Antimicrob Agents Chemother*. 2002; **46**: 2238–43.

[13.10.4] Dimeticone (OTC)

Class:	surface-acting silicone polymer
Lotion:	dimeticone 4%
Dose:	**for head lice**
	adults and children over 6 months (unlicensed use under 6 months): rub into dry hair and scalp, allow to dry naturally, shampoo after 8 h (or overnight); repeat application after 1 week
Pack:	50, 150 mL
Side-effects:	local irritation
Interactions:	none
Cautions:	flammable
Selection:	unlike conventional insecticides, dimeticone works in a physical way, coating the lice and thus preventing excess water being excreted. Thus resistance to chemically acting parasiticides is not a problem. Dimeticone is less of an irritant than alternative treatments

References

Burgess IF. The mode of action of dimeticone 4% lotion against head lice, *Pediculus capitis*. *BMC Pharmacol*. 2009; **9**: 3.

Burgess IF, Brown CM, Lee PN. Treatment of head louse infestation with 4% dimeticone lotion: randomised controlled equivalence trial. *BMJ*. 2005; **330**: 1423.

[13.10.4] Malathion (OTC)

Class: organophosphorus parasiticidal

Liquid: malathion 0.5% in an aqueous base

Dose: **for head lice**

adults and children over 6 months (unlicensed use under 6 months): rub into dry hair and scalp, allow to dry naturally, shampoo after 12 h; comb the hair, ideally with a fine toothed metal comb; repeat application after 1 week

Pack: 50, 200 mL

Side-effects: rarely skin irritation

Interactions: none

Cautions: avoid contact with eyes, broken or infected skin. Avoid repeated doses at intervals less than 1 week or for more than 3 consecutive weeks

Selection: if dimeticone fails when treating head lice, then the next option is malathion, which is one of the least toxic organophosphorus parasiticides because it is rapidly inactived by an enzyme in human plasma

References

Burgess IF. Head lice. *Clin Evid (Online)*. 2011; pii: 1703.

Tebruegge M, Pantazidou A, Curtis N. What's bugging you? An update on the treatment of head lice infestation. *Arch Dis Child Educ Pract Ed*. 2011; **96**: 2–8.

[13.10.4] Permethrin dermal cream (OTC)

Class: pyrethroid parasiticidal for treatment of scabies

Cream: permethrin 5%

Dose: **for scabies**

adults and children over 2 months: apply over the whole skin surface, do not wash hands after treatment (if any part is washed, then reapply permethrin to the area afterwards), wash off after 8–12 h, repeat after 7 days. Prescribe sufficient to treat all members of the household simultaneously, each application needing:

adults: 30 g

children 6–12 years: 15 g

1–5 years: 7 g

2 months–1 year: 4 g

Pack: 30 g

Side-effects: itching, redness, stinging; rarely rashes, oedema

Interactions: none

Cautions: not for children under 2 months; avoid contact with eyes, broken or infected skin. Ensure you prescribe the 5% strength, not the 1% cream rinse preparation, which would be inadequate. Ingested permethrin is toxic, so in young children and anyone who is debilitated or confused it is also necessary to avoid the vicinity of the mouth, where it could be licked off

Selection: permethrin cream, in an aqueous base, is suitable for everyone, including young children, and people with asthma or eczema. Only about 0.5% of the applied permethrin is absorbed and that is rapidly metabolised. Malathion is a suitable non-pyrethroid parasiticidal alternative

Reference

Strong M, Johnstone PW. Interventions for treating scabies. *Cochrane Database Syst Rev.* 2007; 3: CD000320.

Borderline Substances

[A2.3.1] SMA LF

Class:	specialised formula enteral feed
Infant feed:	low lactose
Pack:	430 g
Selection:	use for up to 6 weeks as part of a low-lactose diet in babies with persistent diarrhoea after gastro-enteritis

Reference

Stanley S. *Guidance on the Treatment of Gastroenteritis*. Report for the Sheffield Teaching Hospitals Foundation Trust, Appendix 4; 2008. Available at: www.sheffield.nhs.uk/professionals/resources/infantfeeding/apps.pdf (accessed 17 September 2011).

13

Resources

Reference books

British National Formulary (BNF) – updated every 6 months and published by the BMA and Royal Pharmaceutical Society of Great Britain. Also available online at http://bnf.org. Make sure you are not using an out-of-date copy! Instead, give it to Pharmaid (Tel: 020 7572 2364, admin@commonwealthpharmacy.org).

OTC Directory – published annually by the Proprietary Society of Great Britain. Details (and pictures) of many common over-the-counter preparations. Obtain the book from www.pagb. co.uk/publications/otcdirectory.html or look online at www.medicinechestonline.com

Other reading

Ashton R, Leppard B. *Differential Diagnosis in Dermatology*. Oxford: Radcliffe; 2004. ISBN: 1-85775-660-6.

Fry J, Sandler G. *Common Diseases: their nature, prevalence and care*. 5th ed. Amsterdam: Kluwer Academic; 1993. ISBN: 978-0-7923-8803-6.

Greenstein B, Gold D. *Trounce's Clinical Pharmacology for Nurses*. 18th ed. Edinburgh: Churchill Livingstone; 2008. ISBN: 978-0-443-06804-1.

Guillebaud J. *Contraception: your questions answered*. 5th ed. Edinburgh: Churchill Livingstone; 2008. ISBN: 978-0-443-06908-6.

Neal MJ. *Medical Pharmacology at a Glance*. 6th ed. Hoboken, NJ: Wiley-Blackwell; 2009. ISBN: 978-1-4051-8197-6.

Rushforth H. *Assessment Made Incredibly Easy*. UK edition. Lippincott, Williams & Wilkins; 2009. ISBN: 978-1-901831-07-8.

Phone

FPA helpline for sexual health and contraceptive advice. England: 0845 122 8690, Northern Ireland: 0845 122 8687

Online

www.minorillness.co.uk: our own website

This book contains a voucher which will give you 6 months' free access to the members' section, with online educational materials and email alerts.

Scan this QR code with your smartphone to take you there directly.

http://prodigy.clarity.co.uk: the most useful site for detailed, evidence-based advice on minor illness

www.patient.co.uk: a good source of patient information leaflets and self-help groups

www.evidence.nhs.uk: many useful resources, including the *BNF* and the Cochrane Library

www.tripanswers.org: for the answer to that awkward question

www.labtestsonline.org: for advice about laboratory tests

www.dermnetnz.org: for skin conditions

www.hpa.org.uk: for information on infectiousness and school exclusion

www.dh.gov.uk/en/Publichealth/Immunisation/index.htm: current immunisation schedules and the 'Green Book' *Immunisation Against Infectious Disease* (original version 1996, many new chapters available online)

www.spottingthesickchild.com: detailed advice on the examination of children

www.nice.org.uk: national guidance on a wide range of conditions

www.nathnac.org: travel advice

www.travax.scot.nhs.uk: up-to-date advice about travel vaccination and malaria

www.dwp.gov.uk/fitnote: information about MED3 certificates

www.bashh.org: information and guidelines on sexual health

http://ukpmc.ac.uk: for free access to millions of publications

All websites listed here were accessed 2 May 2011.

Prescribing information sources

Internet resources

Many of the best and most up-to-date information sources are on the internet, either freely available or available with an NHS Athens password via **www.evidence.nhs.uk**

Source	Website
British National Formulary	http://bnf.org
OTC drug information	www.pagb.co.uk
Electronic Medicines Compendium	www.medicines.org.uk Patient information leaflet (PIL) and Summary of product characteristics (SPC), including frequencies of side-effects and half-life
Monthly Index of Medical Specialities	www.mims.co.uk Pharmaceutically sponsored, but has a useful table of emollient additives
The Cochrane Library	www.thecochranelibrary.com
PubMed medical database	www.ncbi.nlm.nih.gov/pubmed
Bandolier	www.medicine.ox.ac.uk/bandolier
National Prescribing Centre	www.npc.co.uk Type in 'common infections' and try the quizzes. Also see the non-medical prescribers' section
UK Medicines Information Central	www.ukmicentral.nhs.uk Prescribing information for breastfeeding mothers

Abbreviations

5-HT	5-hydroxytryptamine
ACEI	angiotensin-converting enzyme inhibitor
ADR	adverse drug reaction
BDI-II	Beck Depression Inventory II
BP	blood pressure
BTS	British Thoracic Society
BV	bacterial vaginosis
CCG	clinical commissioning group
CD	controlled drug
COC	combined oral contraceptive
COPD	chronic obstructive pulmonary disease
CRT	capillary refill time
DMARD	disease-modifying anti-rheumatic drugs
EC	emergency contraception
e/c	enteric-coated
ECG	electrocardiogram
eGFR	estimated glomerular filtration rate
ENT	Ear, Nose and Throat
ESR	erythrocyte sedimentation rate
FBC	full blood count
FBG	fasting blood glucose
G6PD	glucose-6-phosphate dehydrogenase
GI	gastrointestinal
HADS	Hospital Anxiety and Depression Scale
HPA	Health Protection Agency
HPU	Health Protection Unit
HRT	hormone replacement therapy
HVS	high vaginal swab
IUCD	intrauterine contraceptive device
IUS	intrauterine system
IV	intravenous
LMP	last menstrual period
MAOI	monoamine oxidase inhibitor
MDI	metered dose inhaler
MMR	measles, mumps and rubella
m/r	modified-release
MRSA	methicillin-resistant *Staphylococcus aureus*

MSU	mid-stream urine
NICE	National Institute for Health and Clinical Excellence
NIP	nurse independent prescriber
NMC	Nursing and Midwifery Council
NMIC	National Minor Illness Centre
OTC	over the counter
PCT	primary care trust
PHQ-9	Patient Health Questionnaire 9
POP	progestogen-only pill
PPI	proton pump inhibitor
RR	respiratory rate
SHA	strategic health authority
SIGN	Scottish Intercollegiate Guidelines Network
SSRI	selective serotonin reuptake inhibitor
STI	sexually transmitted infection
TENS	transcutaneous electrical nerve stimulation
UPSI	unprotected sexual intercourse
URTI	upper respiratory tract infection
ZIG	zoster immunoglobulin

Index

NOTE: entries in **bold** refer to boxes, figures and tables.